A Nurse's Survival Guide to Leadership and Management on the Ward

At Elsevier, we understand the importance of providing up-to-date and relevant content. For this reason, we are continuously working on updated editions and new titles for the series. Please visit our website to find out the latest news and the upcoming publications: https://www.uk.elsevierhealth.com/.

A Nurse's Survival Guide to Leadership and Management on the Ward

Third Edition

Brian Dolan, OBE, FRSA, MSc (Oxon), MSc (Nurs), RMN, RGN
Director, Health Service 360; Visiting Professor of Nursing, Oxford
Institute of Nursing, Midwifery and Allied Health Research
(OxINMAHR), Oxford;
Honorary Professor of Leadership in Healthcare, Salford University,
Director of Service Improvement, Canterbury District Health Board,
New Zealand

Amy Overend, FRSA, RGN, DiPHE, QIS
Neonatal Intensive Care Specialist Sister, Royal Bolton NHS Foundation
Trust, Farnworth, Bolton, UK
Trustee & Non-Executive Director at Bliss; NHS Assembly Committee
Member; NIHR Expert Reviewer

ELSEVIER

First edition 2006
Second edition 2013

The rights of Brian Dolan and Amy Overend to be identified as authors of this work has been asserted by them in accordance with the Copyright, Designs and Patents Act 1988.

Notices

ISBN: 978-0-7020-7662-6

Printed in United Kingdom

Last digit is the print number: 9 8 7 6 5 4 3

Content Strategist: Poppy Garraway/Serena Castelnovo
Content Development Specialist: Kirsty Guest
Project Manager: Janish Ashwin Paul
Design: Amy Buxton

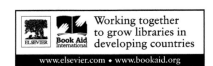

Working together
to grow libraries in
developing countries

www.elsevier.com • www.bookaid.org

Contents

Dedications

My family and friends care for and about me, challenge my thinking and make each day a blessing. I am constantly grateful in a life that traverses the United Kingdom, Ireland, New Zealand and Australia and somehow works because of everyone's support. Thank you and I love and appreciate you all more than you can ever know.

Thank you to Professor Jane Cummings, a loyal and treasured friend over many years, a remarkable Chief Nursing Officer for England (2012–18), and sponsor for my #EndPJparalysis and #Last1000days campaigns to value patient time. Through her unwavering support, what was a whisper among colleagues became a powerful international chorus and for that, and so many acts of personal and professional kindness, I will always be grateful.

Finally, I dedicate this book to my beloved friend, mentor and counsel, Professor Janet Marsden FRCN (1961–2018). A global giant in ophthalmic nursing, co-creator of the internationally acclaimed Manchester Triage System, an exceptionally original thinker and a passionate educator, leader and manager. Janet is deeply missed by all of us who were so very fortunate enough to know her. To translate the apt Irish saying 'Ní bheidh sí leithéidí ann arís' – 'Her likes will not be seen again'.

Brian Dolan

First of all, I dedicate this book to my wonderful sister Megan, who is always my loudest and most steadfast supporter of all that I do. Without her unwavering support, even in the hardest of times, I would not be where I am today, both personally and professionally. She is my rock, my inspiration and who I aspire to be like every single day, and no thank you will ever be enough.

To the amazing people in my life who continuously support me, even when I doubt myself, thank you. Your continuous confidence, love and support for me shine through, and I am exceptionally lucky to have you in my life; you make me a better human.

Finally, to my colleagues – you are the most amazing team and our patients are so incredibly lucky to have you looking after them. Thank you for all that you do!

Amy Overend

Foreword

Even as a student nurse in Southmead Hospital, Bristol, in 1980, where I had enthusiastically started my training in September 1979, I was very aware of the importance of a publication by the distinguished Dr. Sue Pembrey, which was based on her PhD work with 50 – what we knew in those days as – Ward Sisters. This seminal work was titled *The Ward Sister: Key to Nursing* (Pembrey 1980) and it had three important messages:

Good nursing care does not just happen but needs to be organised as a deliberate management function;

Ward Sisters need to be able to exercise control and authority in order to coordinate the services necessary to ensure individualised care;

Ward Sisters identified learnt behaviours from observing the practice of other more senior sisters articulating the need for strong role models in practice.

Dr. Pembrey, who was recently named as one of the 70 most influential nurses and midwives who helped shaped the NHS (Royal College of Nursing Institute, 2018), reported that due to the size and complexity of their role, many of the Ward Sisters failed to fully understand what the role encompassed and had experienced a distinct lack of preparation before commencing their post.

Her findings are as pertinent today as they were during her research 40 years ago – particularly in that Ward Sisters required being highly educated, able to teach, manage and lead a team of staff.

While it may be nearly 40 years since Dr. Pembrey's work, and the context in which we deliver health and care has changed almost beyond recognition, the need to have highly educated Ward Managers/Team Leaders – which is the much more appropriate modern title now – who can teach, motivate, lead and inspire their teams has not changed in the slightest – wherever they work – be it in an in-patient, primary care, community or social care setting.

When I was appointed as Chief Nursing Officer (CNO) for England in 2012 and thought about my own career trajectory, it gave me the opportunity to remind colleagues that sometimes we may be at risk momentarily of looking back through some rose-tinted spectacles and thinking that professional life may have been a little better in the past. We may think that practising as a nurse may then have seemed more straightforward, less political and pressurised – however, when truly remembering things like being left solely as a third year student in charge of a busy and complex ward – I am aware of how much the profession has grown and adapted into the attractive and rewarding career it is today – and that the negative and quite frankly risky experiences should no longer occur.

I am also passionate about identifying what is better today, while not forgetting to take the best of where we have come from. This has been a constant mantra in my career that has taken me from a variety of roles such as Staff Nurse, Sister, Clinical Nurse Specialist, Director of Nursing and the pinnacle of my career to serve for nearly seven years as CNO. I see these principles as the linchpin for improving patient outcomes and experience, staff well-being and the delivery of safe and effective care.

It is why I first developed and introduced the six Cs in 2012 – Care, Compassion, Competence, Communication, Courage and Commitment at the beginning of my tenure as CNO (NHS England 2012). I strongly believed that they were a way to articulate the values of nursing and foster conversations about what matters. The aligned *Compassion in Practice* strategy set out our shared purpose as nurses, midwives and care staff to deliver high-quality, compassionate care, and to achieve excellent health and well-being outcomes.

Building on that, I launched *Leading Change, Adding Value* in May 2016 (NHS England 2016), as a framework for nursing, midwifery and care staff to support transformational change across the system. Everyone is a leader, no matter where they work or what they do, and the framework demonstrates the capability, contribution and leadership of nursing, midwifery and care staff across the health and care sectors to narrowing the three gaps in the Five Year Forward View.

While change may be constant in nursing, the values, the expertise, the desire to help others and make it better remain undimmed and I am certain that nursing's voice, influence and position is stronger than ever. Being a Ward Manager/Team Leader involves lots of work but is an amazing opportunity that enables you to guide, develop and inspire others.

For those starting out on the journey of being such a leader, I wish you well and you stand on the shoulders of generations of nurses and midwives before you. It is a great place to be in a profession, I am proud to have joined almost four decades ago.

Professor Jane Cummings, Chief Nursing Officer for England (2012–18).

References

Royal College of Nursing Institute, 2018. 70 NHS Years: A Celebration of 70 Influential Nurses and Midwives from 1948 to 2018. RCNi, London.

NHS England, 2013. Compassion in Practice: Nursing, Midwifery and Care Staff. Our Vision and Strategy. NHS England, London.

NHS England, 2016. Leading Changing, Adding Value: A Framework for Nurses, Midwives and Care Staff. NHS England, London.

Pembrey, S., 1980. The Ward Sister - Key to Nursing: Study of the Organisation of Individualised Nursing. Royal College of Nursing, London.

Preface to Third Edition

Nursing may simply be a practice, but it is a practice that is far from simple. For those starting out on their journey to ward/unit leadership and management, it may seem a practice that is mysterious and full of new jargon, ways of working and even thinking.

A nurses's guide to leadership and management on the ward originally saw light under the authorship of Jenny Thomas in 2006 and 2013, and we wish to acknowledge her work. In that time, while the underpinning values of role modelling, inspiring and motivating may not have changed, the context in which staff practice and are led has altered dramatically both organisationally and culturally. No longer is it enough to expect respect, demand control and insist on authority; the nursing world has become a much less hierarchical, more complex place; and approximately 70% of the book has been completely rewritten for this third edition.

We have retained most of Thomas' chapters as they remain relevant to being able to survive and thrive as a ward/unit manager; being clear about roles and responsibilities, prioritising work, creating a positive environment, recruitment, managing staff and budgets, being politically aware, being a good role model etc. Some things do not and should not change when it comes to doing the job.

Indeed, it could have been nursing that Michael Oakshott, the philosopher and political theorist, was talking about when he described education as 'a transaction between the generations'. We subscribe to that view although we would probably have called education 'a mutually respectful conversation between the generations! The importance of learning from the wisdom of others who have gone before and those who follow behind, recognising that teams are built on trust, that kindness matters a lot and that it is better to have influence than power is a philosophy to life and work we both share.

As authors, we have both worked as unit managers for years in adult and neonatal intensive care (Overend) and emergency departments (Dolan) and have experienced the many highs and lows that come with the role. Knowing we made a difference, however small, each day to patients and staff has made the challenges worthwhile even while acknowledging our own learning and constant need to keep growing as managers and leaders every day. Leadership and management on the ward/unit is a journey without end, always striving to make it better for patients and staff alike.

The first edition of this book was not the start of the conversation about ward/unit leadership and management, nor will this edition complete it. What we hope this book will provide you with is the tools to become an even better ward/unit manager and leader, to further build your confidence in yourself and your team and enable you to share what you have learnt, so others will stand on your shoulders as they succeed themselves.

This book continues a conversation that is far from simple in practice but one that we believe remains a crucial endeavour and more important than ever for the profession we love so much.

Brian Dolan and Amy Overend
October 2018

Preface to Second Edition

The role of ward manager is so important yet so overlooked in today's health-care system. Unfortunately, the role has become so huge that some are struggling to keep up with the day-to-day demands of running shifts and completing all the paperwork, leaving little time or energy left to lead nursing. There are few specific training programmes, which means that learning often takes place through trial and error. This is not the most effective way to build up the skills and confidence required to lead. In addition, it is a rather isolated role at a time when support is probably most needed in your career.

I spent many years as a ward manager, yet it was not until I reached senior manager/deputy director level that I finally found out the things I should have known back then. No one told me how to run a budget; I just started receiving budget statements each month. No one told me how to investigate and write a complaint response; I simply assumed that what I did was right because no one told me otherwise. In fact, I still did not know the proper procedure until I spent a year afterwards working in a complaints department. I attended numerous management courses and learnt about various management theories and models, but few gave specific information on how to do things in real life. I still picked up most of my job through experience – not ideal.

I now provide teaching programmes, facilitate workshops and support groups for ward managers and matrons and have been asked many times which book I got my information from. But there was no book. Most of the content in this book is taken from nearly 30 years of personal experience and observations. I gained a lot of this information from all the jobs I have had in healthcare *since* being a ward manager.

This book differs from other management and leadership books in that it is a practical guide; it is not an academic book. It is written in everyday language, specifically avoiding management jargon and academic theories. It also includes tips on how to cut through red tape and bureaucracy and put the patient first.

This is basically a 'how-to' book. When you need to look up how to do something, the last thing you need to do is wade through lots of academic theory. You will find this book helpful whether you are planning to be a ward manager, have recently taken on the role or even if you have many years of experience in the role. Matrons will also find it a useful guide for teaching and developing their teams. Although the book is aimed specifically at ward managers, it can be applied to clinical managers of any setting, including A&E, ICU and outpatients.

This second edition has been updated to reflect the current healthcare environment which has changed markedly over the past few years. There is a greater focus on achieving set performance/quality indicators with the added pressure of delivering a more effective service for less cost. There are tips throughout the book on dealing with these pressures while ensuring that care remains patient centred and you and your staff do not burn yourselves out trying to deliver the impossible. The increased focus on learning from our mistakes and being open about them has been taken into account with the addition of a new chapter which takes you through the current guidance on 'Improving quality and safety'.

The first eight chapters concentrate on the basic skills required for the ward manager's role. The next few Chapters 9–12 give information on how to be more effective in your role. And finally, Chapters 13–15 discuss common problems for ward managers, suggested solutions and where to go for the most appropriate advice.

This book can be easily read through from cover to cover. It contains useful action points at the end of each chapter, which you may wish to use to inform your personal development plan. It can also be used as a handy reference book in times of need. You can look up quickly how to deal with an allegation of bullying, for example, or how to calculate your team's study leave allowance.

Although the content of the book is mainly based in the context of the NHS, it is also relevant for those working in private healthcare. Most private healthcare companies base their policies and procedures on at least those required within the NHS sector. In England, all private providers have been required to register with the Care Quality Commission since April 2011 and are therefore subject to the same care standard regulations as NHS organisations.

I hope you enjoy reading this book and that it provides you with the support and practical information you need to do the job effectively and to keep yourself sane in what must be one of the most difficult and demanding jobs within healthcare.

London 2011
Jenny Thomas

About the Author

Jenny Thomas has worked in healthcare for nearly 30 years including several years as a ward manager, matron/senior nurse and deputy director of nursing. She has considerable experience in supporting and developing ward managers and matrons and still works with these groups as a senior lecturer at London South Bank University. She holds academic and professional qualifications in nursing, management and education.

Chapter 1

The Role of the Ward Manager

1.1 INTRODUCTION

When you become a nurse manager your responsibilities change. Most of your education and experience to date will have been focused on clinical practice, but the manager's role requires a very different set of skills. You are required to manage a team of staff with a set budget and are responsible for maintaining an environment in which people can work well.

Being a good nurse does not necessarily mean that you are naturally a good nurse manager. The two roles are very distinct. As a nurse, you are responsible for providing patients with a high standard of care. As a nurse manager, you are responsible for providing patients with a high standard of care *through others*. It takes time and experience to learn the art of being a good manager. Clarifying exactly what is expected of you in your role is the first major step.

1.2 BE CLEAR ABOUT WHAT 24-H RESPONSIBILITY MEANS

Ward managers carry 24-h responsibility for the ward. This means you are required to ensure that systems and processes are in place for patients to receive a high standard of care from your team, day and night, irrespective of whether you are there or not. It also means that you could be liable for poor patient care when you are not there if it is evident that you did not do everything to ensure that those systems and processes were in place. This includes:

- the appropriate development and support of your staff;
- appropriate policies, guidelines and standards;
- adequate rosters;
- sufficient risk management activities.

The individual nurses in your team are registered professionals and therefore responsible and accountable for their own actions or inactions, under the terms of their registration. However, as their manager, you may be liable if you do not provide the right working conditions for your team to provide good care. You are also responsible and accountable for healthcare assistants who are based on your ward, are managed directly or indirectly by you and who deliver direct patient care. The same principle applies for ward clerks and the key is having the confidence and assurance that those who you manage do so to standards that meet the organisation's and legal minimum standards.

1.3 UNLESS IT IS AN EMERGENCY, DISCOURAGE BEING CALLED AT HOME

The term '24-h responsibility' does not mean that you should be accessible out of hours. It is a common misconception that the ward manager should be available at all times. There have been instances when on-call or site managers have called ward managers at home or on their mobile phones to sort out issues and it is unwise to encourage it. Home distractions or tiredness could also impair your response.

It is different if you have not done your job properly. For example, if some staff do not turn up for work on your ward one day and it is not clear on the roster who should be working that shift, then that is your responsibility. It means that you did not ensure adequate cover in your absence, and therefore need to be contacted to clarify matters. However, if members of your staff call in sick when you are not there, leaving shifts uncovered, it is the responsibility of the shift leader, matron or site manager to deal with the problem.

It is also not appropriate for members of your own team to be calling you at home. Your role is to enable them to make their own decisions and not to have to call you out of hours for advice. It is the responsibility of both you and your organisation to ensure that other senior managers are there to turn to for advice and support in emergencies when you are not there. This is usually the matron during office hours and some sort of on-call or site manager out of hours. If there is no such system properly in place, you could be liable for failing to address this omission.

1.4 MINIMISING RISK

Having 24-h responsibility for your ward means you must minimise the risk of anything untoward happening in your absence by ensuring that:

- the appropriate health and safety procedures are in place;
- the appropriate resources are available, including staff;
- all members of your team have full access and have been made aware of all the appropriate policies and guidelines to inform them of the standards expected;
- all members of your team have had appropriate induction and ongoing development to ensure they are competent in their role.

1.5 YOUR PROFESSIONAL AND MANAGERIAL ACCOUNTABILITY

The Nursing and Midwifery Council (NMC) does not offer any specific guidance on the accountability of nurse managers. However, it does include the aspect of being accountable for how and when to delegate. The NMC code (NMC, 2015a,b) requires that, when delegating, you must:

- only delegate tasks and duties that are within the other person's scope of competence, making sure that they fully understand your instructions;

- make sure that everyone you delegate tasks to is adequately supervised and supported so they can provide safe and compassionate care; and
- confirm that the outcome of any task you have delegated to someone else meets the required standard.

In 2002, one of the reasons for removing a matron from the register was cited as placing 'unreasonable demands on staff'. A unit manager was also removed for 'failing to take appropriate action when a member of staff assaulted a patient'. In other words, as a manager who is also an NMC registrant, you are failing to uphold the code if you do not put the interests of the patients first in any managerial decisions that you make. This is also made clear in the code of conduct for NHS managers (Department of Health, 2002), which states that 'the care and safety of patients' should be your first concern and you must 'act to protect them from risk'.

1.6 RAISING CONCERNS

If you are working under extreme pressure or there are staffing shortages out of your control, you must report it to the appropriate senior manager and be able to demonstrate that you have made every effort to remedy the situation. Again, this is made clear in Section 16 of the NMC Code (2015a,b) which also adds that you should 'acknowledge and act on all concerns raised to you, investigating, escalating or dealing with those concerns where it is appropriate for you to do so' (NMC, 2015a,b).

You should also be alert to pressures being felt by your staff, since over-worked staff may act inappropriately. In 2011, the NMC found 'basically a good nurse' with 'no evidence of general incompetence' who was 'dedicated to a career in nursing' guilty of misconduct when she failed to summon assistance or commence resuscitation on a pulseless patient and completed the patient's fluid charts retrospectively. In another case, the High Court held that the NMC had been unduly lenient in not finding unfitness to practice on the part of a midwife who failed to provide support to a junior colleague undergoing preceptorship and subsequently spoke in a bullying and intimidatory manner towards the person who had reported her. It is important to raise concerns over staff pressures rather than raise your voice to staff.

The NMC has produced clear guidelines for raising concerns to help all nurses and midwives (NMC, 2015a,b) and the Royal College of Nursing (RCN) has produced some guidelines that are particularly relevant for ward managers and shift nurses in charge (RCN, 2009, 2017). These guidelines also detail what you should include when raising your concerns in writing, such as:

- evidencing your concerns
- being specific
- identifying actions that you have already taken
- being precise about exactly what is needed to remedy the situation
- asking for an acknowledgement of your concern

If your line manager fails to address your concern, then you should raise it with your organisation's designated person. Every organisation is required to have a designated person with specific training and responsibility for dealing with escalated concerns. For nurses and midwives, it is usually (but not always) the director of nursing. Only ever consider taking your concerns further (e.g. regulatory organisation, MP or media) once you have exhausted these routes within your own organisation, and never do so until you have sought advice from the NMC, RCN or other trade union. Public Concern at Work is an independent charity that also offers free advice in such situations (www.pcaw.co.uk).

1.6.1 Be Clear About What Makes a Good Leader

Your job title is a 'manager'; however, this does not automatically make you a good leader. Your job is to manage staff and resources to ensure that patients on your ward receive a good standard of care. If you lead well, your job as a manager will be far easier. The difference between a manager and a leader is this: a manager does things right, whereas a leader gets the right things done, most often through others; the best do both. Good leaders also enable their team to question whether the things need doing in the first place.

There are various leadership models promoted within healthcare, the most common being transformational and shared (or distributed) leadership.

1.7 TRANSFORMATIONAL LEADERSHIP

Transformational leadership is about influencing others to do things. The transformational leader is often charismatic and inspirational, and they are more considerate towards individuals. They stimulate people to be more creative and to challenge the system if necessary. Boamah et al. (2018) argue that managers who demonstrate transformational leadership in the workplace have greater potential to create environments that support professional nursing practice that promote high-quality patient care. The opposite of transformational is transactional. Transactional leadership applies to the older managerial style of setting tasks, giving rewards to those who achieve them and 'punishing' those who do not.

It is debatable as to whether transformational leadership is the model that is actually being used throughout practice at the moment, or whether it is entirely appropriate, since the emphasis on meeting performance indicators can be viewed as largely transactional. However, a transformational leader will not only ask their team how indicators can be met, they will also question them and look at alternative solutions if they are detrimental to the overall patient care. A transformational leader may also help shape the language, so staff do not think of them as targets, with all the perceived transactional negativity that can be associated with that, and instead speak of internal professional standards that the team should aspire to meet. So even in a transactional organisation, you can be transformational in your approach.

To become more transformational in your style, it would be worth considering the five practices of good leadership based on 30 years of research by Kouzes and Posner (2017). These are to:

- inspire a shared vision
- model the way
- challenge the process
- encourage the heart
- enable others to act

1.7.1 Inspire a Shared Vision

Leaders are driven by a sense of what is possible and what their unit can become. Get the team together and ask them about where they all want to be in the future, or more realistically in a year's time. Then work backwards in 180, 90, 60 and 30 day blocks to facilitate them to set specific objectives together that they are all willing to work towards. Leaders believe they can make a difference and give others the belief and confidence to do the same.

1.7.2 Model the Way

The most important personal quality people look for and admire in a leader is credibility because if people do not believe in the messenger they will not believe in their message. Set an example about the standards you want your team to achieve and give them regular individual feedback about their progress. This means spending time with them, sharing experiences where your values come alive and asking questions that help them focus on values and priorities. Show them how to cut through the bureaucracy and/or be the person who cuts it for them.

1.7.3 Challenge the Process

The real work of leaders is change, and no one has ever been a successful leader by keeping things the same. Continually question and look for ways of improving care in your ward. Encourage your staff to question decisions made by others, including other health professionals, by having the appropriate knowledge, confidence and support in order to do so. Encourage them also to challenge you; a leader embraces challenges with grace and is not hidebound by hierarchy or title; they seek challenge everywhere to be a better leader.

1.7.4 Encourage the Heart

Leaders tend to be positive and optimistic, even in challenging times as they recognise both positivity and negativity (especially) are infectious. Pay attention to what matters to individuals and personalise appreciation. Encouraging the heart is how leaders visibly and behaviourally link rewards with performance and behaviour with cherished values.

1.7.5 Enable Others to Act

Leadership is very much a team effort and teamwork; trust and empowerment liberate staff to take informed risks. If staff feel their leader has their back, they will flourish, and here trust is critical, as a team without trust is not a team but a group of staff who are co-located in a workplace. Enable and trust your staff to make important decisions and take risks by investing in their development and support. Power is not something to be hoarded but given away in the service of others.

1.8 DEVELOPING PEOPLE – IMPROVING CARE

This is an evidence-based national framework to guide action on improvement skill-building, leadership development and talent management for people (NHS Improvement, 2016). The overall aim of the framework is 'Continuous improvement in care for people, population health and value for money'. The five conditions (primary drivers) are:

1. Leaders equipped to develop high-quality local health and care systems in partnership;
2. Compassionate, inclusive and effective leaders at all levels;
3. Knowledge of improvement methods and how to use them at all levels;
4. Support systems for learning at local, regional and national levels;
5. Enabling, supportive and aligned regulation and oversight.

Various development programmes which offer online and/or face-to-face content are available for ward managers through the NHS Leadership Academy, whose courses such as the Edward Jenner and Mary Seacole programmes are excellent for those starting in leadership roles. The King's Fund, RCN and others also offer a range of leadership programmes too.

1.9 SHARED LEADERSHIP

In the mid-2000s, there were major enquiries into leadership, care, governance and quality standards over a number of years at Maidstone and Tunbridge Wells NHS Foundation Trust where outbreaks of *Clostridium difficile* led to at least 90 deaths (Healthcare Commission, 2007), and Mid Staffordshire NHS Foundation Trust, where at least 400 more patients than would be expected died (Department of Health, 2013). Each enquiry clearly showed failures in leadership, not only at the top of these organisations but throughout, as clinicians felt powerless to do anything; however, it should not absolve clinicians from responsibility either. Scandals such as these have highlighted the need for all clinicians to be leaders and develop the skills to take action in such situations. Shared leadership is about all healthcare staff being able to see what needs doing or what needs to change and having the skills to work with others in order to do it. Clinicians should develop the leadership skills to work in partnership with experienced non-clinical managers and vice versa.

If you make decisions that affect your staff or patients based on the advice of one person alone, you cannot blame them if your decision was the wrong one. If there is a serious incident, for example, and you take a course of action that your manager advised, you may remain responsible for the outcome of that decision, just as your staff must make informed decisions about their own practice rather than relying solely on you. Leadership and management is a team sport so get advice from others as well before you make decisions, so they are informed by different perspectives.

1.10 YOUR LINE MANAGER

Your line manager will not be your only source of advice as not all line managers have been ward managers and know what the role entails. And of those who have had experience, how can you be sure that their experience is any better than yours and that they are giving you the right advice?

Sometimes nurses rely too heavily on the next person above them within the hierarchical system. This can be a mistake as being more senior does not necessarily mean that you have more relevant experience. That is not to say you should ignore the advice and guidance of your line manager as there are many very good and experienced matrons and service managers. However, it is always advisable to seek guidance from a variety of sources so that you can make an informed choice.

1.11 YOUR MENTOR

As a ward manager, it can be very helpful to find yourself a mentor, usually someone senior in the organisation. Mentors can be used as a sounding board to expand your knowledge and skills, gain valuable advice from a more experienced person and build professional networks. Most board or assistant board directors are keen to mentor someone from the clinical setting within their own organisation. A senior manager from another hospital or even a non-healthcare setting can be advantageous, as they will often have a different perspective (see Chapter 10 for further information on mentorship in management).

1.12 YOUR CLINICAL SUPERVISOR

It would also be wise to have a clinical supervisor. You need to have someone who is more experienced than you in your specialist area to help you reflect and learn from your clinical practice. This could be a nurse specialist, consultant doctor/nurse or another more experienced ward manager (see Chapter 5 for further information on clinical supervision).

1.13 THE HUMAN RESOURCES DEPARTMENT

Do not rely solely on your line manager or colleagues for advice regarding personnel issues. If you have problems with staff, such as inappropriate behaviour, sickness/absence problems or incompetence, your HR department will be able to provide the most up-to-date information with which you can then make the most appropriate decision. A meeting with your HR advisor on a monthly basis helps build a good working relationship which will help enormously in times of crisis.

1.14 THE FINANCE DEPARTMENT

If you are going to make any changes at all which may involve extra staff or resources, always consult with your finance advisor first. It is their role to help you calculate the cost of any changes and to advise you what the best course of action is in terms of resources. They can help you become involved in the business planning process for your directorate and you will become far more knowledgeable and effective in accessing appropriate resources. As with HR, you should meet with your finance advisor on a monthly basis.

1.15 OTHER WARD MANAGERS

Another valuable resource often ignored by many ward managers and deputy ward managers is that of other more experienced ward managers. Why do so many ward managers work alone without searching out support from their more experienced peers? If you do not have some sort of group where ward managers get together to share experiences, guide and support each other, it would be a good idea to develop one yourself (see Chapter 10).

Within 3 months of starting your job, request a formal performance review with your manager to clarify your objectives. You should have 3 months first to settle in and identify what needs doing and any further skills that you require to meet those needs.

Your manager will also have specific objective that you are required to fulfil. These usually relate to quality indicators such as the number of complaints, pressure ulcers or infection rates, etc. You may have your own objective such as implementing team nursing, self-rostering or increasing staffing levels. The aim of the performance review is to clarify your objectives together. At your first meeting, you should:

- review where you are now
- agree on your objectives and how these will be achieved
- identify the skills you require to achieve the objectives

A performance review at this stage will ensure that you both agree what your priorities are. There will frequently be more demands than you can meet, and you should work with your manager to prioritise which tasks are more important. You may see that all the patient information leaflets need updating, for example, but if you do not have enough staff to fulfil your minimum staffing requirements, your priority will be to recruit more staff over the next 6 months. Having this set out formally will stop you taking on lots of extra tasks and can stop you working in a different direction to that of your manager.

You should also discuss and understand your line manager's own objectives. Part of your role is to assist your manager in achieving their organisational objectives and you should work together towards the same goals. The performance review process helps to ensure this happens.

1.16 REDUCING THE RISK OF WORK OVERLOAD

Every time you find that there are more things that need to be changed or improved, it can be tempting to go ahead and attempt to add them to your workload. If you feel that your long- and even short- and medium-term priorities need to change, arrange a meeting with your manager to discuss and, if necessary, change your agreed objectives.

Review your progress towards your objectives with your manager regularly. Priorities change frequently, and your objectives should reflect these changes. In addition, frequent reviews help you and your manager understand and appreciate your role and responsibilities.

1.17 FIND OUT WHAT YOU NEED TO KNOW

One challenge with being a ward manager is how do you know what you need to know? How do you know that you are doing the job right? This is especially pertinent if your own manager has never been a ward manager, has only a few years' experience or their experience in the role is limited to one ward only.

This is one of the many reasons why having a wider network is so essential to ensuring you have access to a wider source of knowledge. Take time to set up good links with other ward managers and departments such as HR, finance and facilities. You can use your job description to guide you, or the knowledge and skills framework and build on that assessment. Alternatively, assess yourself using the questionnaire provided in Appendix 1.1. This may help you to identify what you need to know.

1.18 360-DEGREE FEEDBACK

Another way of assessing where you are now is to undertake a 360-degree review. This is an increasingly popular method of gaining feedback from others. It involves filling in a questionnaire assessing yourself against certain criteria and asking your managers, your team and your peers to also fill in the same questionnaire about you and your performance.

You can have a formal 360-degree review through Healthservice 360 (www. healthservice360.co.uk) (which one of the authors, BD, co-directs), the NHS Clinical Leadership Competency Framework or others. Competency-based questionnaires are sent out on your behalf and all the information gathered into a report for you that can include qualitative feedback. You can work through this with a trained facilitator who will help you learn from the report in terms of understanding your strengths and helping you to determine areas that you would like to improve.

1.18.1 Understand Your Legal Responsibilities

NHS Resolution, previously known as the NHS Litigation Authority, is the body charged with addressing legal claims against secondary providers, i.e. hospitals, in the NHS. In 2017/18, the value of payments ran to some £2.23 billion, a 30% increase from £1.71 billion the year before (NHS Resolution, 2018).

Addressing adverse incidents and accusations of negligence cost the NHS a lot of time and money and cause managers and staff immense anxiety. Legal actions can take years to resolve, meaning years of stress. You may have to defend your actions or inactions in court. You may find yourself named repeatedly as the person responsible in a coroner's verdict, which is a public document.

Most nurses are aware of their legal and professional liability for their individual practice. Patients are owed a duty of care by the healthcare organisation and by the individual staff delivering care. The question then is whether that care has been delivered negligently. Ask yourself: What would a reasonable manager do in this situation? What guidelines, protocols or evidence can you produce in justification?

For negligence of any kind to be proved, it must be shown that the following components exist:

- that the defendant (nurse) owed a duty of care to the plaintiff (patient) (established in the case of Donohue v. Stevenson, 1932)
- that the defendant was in breach of that duty (Bolam v. Friern Hospital Management Committee, 1957)
- harm to the plaintiff, which was reasonably foreseeable, resulted directly from the breach of duty of care (Barnett v. Kensington & Chelsea Hospital Management Committee, 1969)

Clinical documentation can be pivotal in cases of negligence (National Audit Office, 2001). The approach that the law tends to take to record-keeping is that if it has not been recorded, it has not been done. It is important staff understand they should be scrupulous in the documentation of their actions to reduce the risk of legal difficulties should a case be brought against them or their colleagues.

1.19 BED MANAGEMENT

As ward manager, you will be liable as a nurse for your personal nursing actions and as a manager you will be liable for your managerial actions. Tensions can arise between the two roles. For instance, pressure on beds might mean frequent requests from the bed management team about patient discharges. To be clear, if a patient is not fit for discharge, they should not be discharged. However, medically fit for discharge is not the same as being nursing or therapeutically fit for discharge, and it is important that the whole multidisciplinary team communicates constantly about the patient's clinical and social status. At a time of growing pressure on beds due to rising demand and an ageing population, it is also incumbent on all staff to ensure patients do not wait in hospital any longer than is necessary for their well-being and that discharge planning meaningfully starts on arrival. Your ward will be one of many in the hospital which is a complex dynamic system so it is important that you and your team remember you are part of a wider team too. The consequences to patients with prolonged waiting for admission from the emergency department are an increased risk of mortality, length of stay and cost (Sun et al., 2013). It is why not declaring beds that have had patients discharged from them should never be acceptable on your ward as it has real effects on patient care and the wider system's effectiveness.

1.20 STAFFING SHORTAGES

Along with funding, and with a shortfall in England alone of some 40,000 nurses, one of the greatest challenges the NHS faces is ensuring safe, adequate staffing day to day, and sometimes it is impossible to get sufficient qualified staff for a shift (RCN, 2009, 2017, 2018). Ensure a proper record is made, submit the appropriate incident form and work with senior managers to find ways to address the problem. In addition to this, you *must* make sure that you make changes to the workload to maintain patient safety. If a patient inadvertently suffers harm in that situation, you should be able to show that as a reasonable, responsible ward manager you met your duty of care.

1.21 SENDING STAFF TO OTHER WARDS

You may be asked to send a member of your team to help on an understaffed ward. You need to consider whether this will put any of your patients at risk. Your duty is towards your own patients; however, it is also about recognising that at hospital level it is a risk-sharing strategy given the pressures on staffing elsewhere. You may also find that members of your staff refuse to go when asked. Listen to the reasons they give and ensure you are not asking them to undertake any responsibility for which they do not have the knowledge or skills. It is better to find out why they refuse to go and identify what would help the situation, such as an agreement with the requesting ward manager on what the member of staff can or cannot do.

1.22 VICARIOUS LIABILITY

Usually, if fault is established, the employing hospital is vicariously liable for the actions of their employees, which means that they pay the compensation to the victim. However, sometimes they can claim all or some of that compensation back from the employee, which happened in the case of Trustees of London Clinic v. Michael Alan Edgar (2001) when a surgeon was held partially liable for nurses' post-operative inactions following a poor handover. The hospital settled out of court but then recovered £30,000 from the surgeon.

1.23 EXPANDED ROLES

Nurses are constantly expanding their roles, and this should be encouraged and welcome; however, your role as manager is to ensure that changes in practice are properly implemented. One Trust agreed that midwives could top up epidurals if trained and assessed as competent by anaesthetists. Over the years, without the Trust realising, this slid into midwives showing other midwives without any formal assessment of competency. An error was made resulting in injury to a patient, and it was held that the midwife was acting outside her scope of practice.

1.24 DUTY TO REPORT CONCERNS REGARDING A STRATEGIC DECISION

Occasionally, a hospital is held to have primary liability. In other words, the hospital's own negligence is the cause of harm. In one case, a hospital decided to employ only one obstetrician at night even though maternity services were on two sites. Lack of timely care meant a twin boy was left brain-damaged even though all the staff present had acted entirely professionally and competently. If a strategic decision by your hospital could put patients at risk, you have a professional duty to report concerns. It should go without saying that whether it is the RCN, Unison or other trade union; it is advantageous to be a member.

1.25 DUTY TO REPORT CAUSES FOR CONCERN REGARDING VULNERABLE PEOPLE

A vulnerable adult is defined as anyone aged 18 years or over 'who is or may be in need of community care services by reason of mental or other disability, age or illness; and who is or may be unable to take care of him or herself, or unable to protect him or herself against significant harm exploitation' (Department of Health, 2000). All such adults that are admitted to your area should be identified and have an appropriate individualised care plan which takes account of their individual needs and circumstances, with the involvement of the person's carer/family.

Vulnerable adults who lack capacity to make their own decisions may need to be protected from harm by measures such as locking ward doors so people with dementia cannot wander off. The Mental Capacity Act 2005 Deprivation of Liberty Safeguards (MCA DOLS) requires all hospitals and care homes to carry out an assessment in such cases to decide whether the care or treatment is being given in a lawful manner. If a person with an MCA DOLS authorisation is transferred from a care home to a hospital and the ward needs to continue to restrict that person's liberty, a fresh MCA DOLS assessment must be carried out.

You must ensure that your team is alert to possible cases of abuse when dealing with vulnerable people. The NMC (2015a,b) notes that abuse or neglect and the different circumstances in which they take place can take many forms. An illustrative list of actions that may constitute neglect or abuse and should give rise to concern includes the following:

- Physical abuse
- Domestic violence
- Sexual abuse
- Psychological abuse
- Financial or material abuse
- Modern slavery
- Discriminatory abuse
- Organisational abuse
- Neglect and acts of omission
- Self-neglect

Ward managers need to be alert to signs of abuse in their patients and also in vulnerable family members, both adults and children. The Office of the Public Guardian (2008) Safeguarding Vulnerable Adults policy includes a comprehensive list of possible indicators of abuse and causal factors (www.publicguardian.gov.uk). If any of your team suspects any type of abuse, they must report it to you, and you must report it promptly to your line manager and follow your local policy for safeguarding vulnerable adults. Remember that staff should record the comments using exactly the same words expressed by the vulnerable adult and should not question them concerning allegations or causes for concern.

There is a duty to refer anyone suspected to have caused harm or pose a risk of harm to a vulnerable adult to the Disclosure and Barring Service (DBS). If you have any concerns, you must raise them with your line manager and ensure they know how to make a referral to the DBS. It is illegal to employ people who are not registered with the DBS to work with vulnerable people.

1.26 SHADOW YOUR MANAGER

It is a good idea to ensure you understand what your manager's role entails, and one way to find out would be to spend some time shadowing your manager. Ask to accompany them to meetings so that you can see for yourself what the job is like and the pressures they are under and how you can support one another to be even better managers and leaders.

1.27 'ACTING UP' IN YOUR MANAGER'S ABSENCE

As you gain experience you may be asked to 'act up' for your line manager to cover for annual leave, sick leave, etc. Make sure you get someone to act up for you too as acting up in someone's absence should not mean carrying on doing your own job as well as covering theirs. Acting up gives you a good insight into the other person's job so ensure you have full responsibility for decision-making and full access to the tools to do the job, e.g. their email, post, agendas for meetings and what you are expected to contribute.

Ensure you have full handover before your manager goes on leave and give a full debrief on their return. You need to know what you did well and what you could have done even better. Doing the same for any members of staff who act up in your absence will also give you insights into their experience of doing your role.

1.28 BUILD UP A GOOD WORKING RELATIONSHIP

Concentrate on building up a good working relationship with your manager. You need to understand their management style, including their preferred mode of communication. You also need to have a good insight into their priorities as well as their stresses and pressures. Part of your role is helping your manager to achieve organisational priorities. Make sure you work with them and not against them. If you do not agree with their decisions, say so constructively ensuring you put across your reasons and offer alternative solutions.

A good healthy working relationship is one in which either of you can challenge the other's decisions constructively without anyone feeling threatened in any way. Always show others that you and your manager work well together and communicate regularly. If people see any stresses and strains in your working relationship, it will reduce their confidence in your management. They need to know that you are both in control.

You need to be able to decipher whether your manager is being reasonable. If you think your manager is not doing things right or is being a bit too bossy, how do you know if that is normal? How do you know that the reason you are not getting the right resources is because they are not putting your case forward in the business plan? The only way you will know is if you understand what their role is and you can also find out from your colleagues. If you maintain good communication with others, you can compare and contrast the role of their managers with yours.

Building up a close working relationship with your manager is so vital for success in your role that this book contains a whole chapter on the subject (see Chapter 12). Knowing and understanding their role is the first step to achieving this aim.

1.28.1 Being the Patients' Advocate

Advocacy is not just about ensuring the patient has the right information and support; it is about influencing a third party on behalf of patients. Your role is to influence others to provide a high standard of care, to protect patients and speak up on their behalf. Participating in committees and networking within the organisation are ways to gain influence and the means to push for change. Connecting through professional bodies and at meetings with colleagues from other organisations can also be helpful in order to learn how those individuals and institutions address similar issues.

1.29 PATIENTS NEED TO FEEL THAT THE MANAGER IS IN CONTROL

Patients and their relatives want someone to ensure that they get good care and that the level of care they get will not depend entirely on whichever individual they get to look after them. They want someone in charge who is able to make decisions and challenge poor practice. They want someone to acknowledge when mistakes are made, ensure they are rectified and that something is done to ensure those mistakes do not happen again.

When a person becomes ill they are at the mercy of those assigned to care for them, and part of your role as the ward manager is to coordinate the healthcare team so the patient receives the best care.

It is not appropriate when a patient or relative makes a complaint to refer them to the complaints.

Where there is a complaint of any kind by a patient or relative, the first action should be to see if it can be resolved quickly, informally and for the most part this is what is done.

In order to act as your patients' advocate, you need to make time to support a direct care process. This gives patients and their relatives confidence that you are:

● supporting the team of nurses
● coordinating with medical and other healthcare professionals
● challenging decisions that may not be appropriate
● ensuring that the focus on performance indicators is not detrimental to the quality of their care
● protecting them from individual incompetence

But most of all they want to be reassured that someone is in charge of the ward and that someone has the time and experience to ensure that they are getting the right care.

1.30 BALANCING YOUR CLINICAL WORK WITH ADMINISTRATIVE DUTIES

Sir Robert Francis, who led the Mid Staffordshire Hospital Inquiry (Department of Health, 2013), made hundreds of recommendations, many of which were germane to nursing, including Recommendation 195:

● Ward nurse managers should operate in a supervisory capacity, and not be office-bound or expected to double up, except in emergencies as part of the nursing provision on the ward.
● They should know about the care plans relating to every patient on his or her ward. They should make themselves visible to patients and staff alike, and be available to discuss concerns with all, including relatives.

- Critically, they should work alongside staff as a role model and mentor, developing clinical competencies and leadership skills within the team.
- As a corollary, they would monitor performance and deliver training and/or feedback as appropriate, including a robust annual appraisal.

The key is to take control of these aspects of your workload. As the ward manager, you could allocate yourself the equivalent of 1 day per week for administrative work. Another option is that you could work the mornings clinically and take 1–2 h each afternoon in the office during the early-late shift overlap. As you gain experience you will increasingly identify what works best for you.

It is certainly not good practice personally or professionally to habitually take work home with you. This is where supportive managers, mentors and colleagues can help so you can draw on their experience and insights on how workloads can be kept as manageable as possible so that the workload does not get taken home or if so is exceptional, not the norm.

1.30.1 Be Aware of the Impact of Your Role on Others

Your style of management not only affects the work of those in your team, it also affects other health professionals who have an input into the care of your patients so it is crucial to ensure that your impact is positive. Wards are often regarded as 'good' or 'bad' depending on who the ward manager is, and this impacts on turnover, staff morale and patient care. While we will deal with this in more detail later in the book, self-awareness of how you come over to others, being able to see the world through the lens of others and being seen as fair and equitable in how you treat everyone matters as everyone notices. As a ward manager you are not off duty for a heartbeat and how you speak to the cleaners or the catering staff will say a lot about you and you will be judged accordingly. Spencer et al. (2014) offer helpful guidance on the transition to ward manager and the dos and don'ts for being a ward manager (Boxes 1.1 and 1.2).

1.31 DOCTORS, ALLIED HEALTH AND OTHER HEALTHCARE PROFESSIONALS

Make the effort to introduce yourself to all new staff, irrespective of their professional background. It does not take much to point out what the routine is, such as how the nursing team works, what is expected of them and what they can expect from you. You and your ward will soon get a good name and they will be more willing to help you if you have proved yourself to be helpful and welcoming in the initial stages.

1.32 NURSING STUDENTS

The way you are perceived in your role is vital to the success of your ward and team. Think back to your student days and your ward placements. What influenced your

Box 1.1 Dos and Don'ts for Ward Managers

Dos

- Plan and prioritise your workload
- Be realistic about what can and cannot be achieved
- Take breaks and ask for help and support
- Reach out and explore the support network (use your peers and support each other)
- Have a clinical supervisor/mentor
- Clarify and review your objectives and skills needed to achieve these
- Work closely with your line manager and understand their management style, priorities and pressures
- Delegate to your deputies, ensuring it is a learning opportunity
- Be proactive and put your ideas forward
- Challenge in the best interests of your patients and staff
- Listen to and support staff, giving them the opportunity to share their ideas
- Give feedback to and motivate your staff
- Always be fair and consistent
- Be approachable
- Have time for staff – always make time to speak to them
- Empower your staff so they can make informed decisions
- Trust your instinct
- Realise you cannot do everything at once
- Be confident to say no when appropriate
- Do not be afraid to have a different opinion
- Involve everyone in your ward
- Remember that it is you who makes a difference

Don'ts

- Allow other people's emergencies to become yours
- Encourage staff to call you at home
- Stay late
- Come in on your day off
- Take work home
- Feel guilty

(From Spencer, C., Al-Sadoon, T., Hemmings, L., Jackson, K., Mulligan, P., 2014. The transition from staff nurse to ward leader. Nursing Times 110 (41), 12–14, reproduced with permission of Nursing Times)

opinion of the experience? Generally, it will have been the ward manager. Many students describe their placement experience in terms of what the ward manager was like. Your influence on others is immense. Be aware that whatever you do or say is under intense scrutiny and will be discussed among students back in the classroom. You cannot afford any students to have 'a bad experience' on your ward. You want your ward to become the one where students want to work once qualified.

In addition to this, role modelling of good patient care and good nursing practice is vital for student development. You must also ensure that students are

Box 1.2 The Transition to Ward Manager

- Applying to be and being appointed as a ward manager
- The joy of wearing the ward manager's uniform and the reaction of colleagues

Novice Ward Manager

- Realising the enormous step from staff nurse to ward manager
- Focussing on the role and fulfiling the job description
- Feeling the weight of expectations – we should know everything
- Learning on the job, dealing with daily challenges of managing staff
- Feeling like the 'new person' in meetings with 'veteran' ward managers
- Finding courage to speak up
- Establishing networks within nursing and multidisciplinary teams
- Spending time with experienced sisters to learn the role
- Finding support from matrons, the head of nursing and the chief nurse

Gaining Confidence

- Establishing a supportive group of managers in a similar position to share problems, thoughts and ideas and to challenge each other
- Using this network to prepare rational arguments for meetings
- Gaining in confidence, finding a voice to speak up

Experienced Ward Manager

- Supporting new ward managers in their roles
- Providing input to training for ward managers including development programmes, human resources and risk management courses

(From Spencer, C., Al-Sadoon, T., Hemmings, L., Jackson, K., Mulligan, P., 2014. The transition from staff nurse to ward leader. Nursing Times 110 (41), 12–14, reproduced with permission of Nursing Times)

not being used to fill ward shortages, so that they have proper opportunities to learn. However, there will be some students who, even with the best support, lack the necessary skills, so you must ensure that your mentors feel confident enough to fail them if necessary (see Chapter 4).

1.33 PATIENTS AND RELATIVES

Patients and relatives will also remember you. They are probably observing you more closely than anyone else. A good habit to get into is to ensure that you speak with every patient every day. While there are various initiatives in place, such as hourly rounding, to ensure their nurse sees all patients, it does make a difference if they see the ward manager each day. It will also help your staff if you can undertake one of their hourly rounds to enable them to pay attention to those patients who really need it.

Make a point of being available at visiting times too. Again, this will be a great support for your staff (enabling them to get on with their work) as well as dealing with the concerns of patients' relatives and carers.

1.34 CONCLUSION

Starting out as a new ward manager can be exciting and terrifying at the same time and it is quite normal to suffer from so-called 'imposter syndrome' where you doubt yourself, your accomplishments and your fitness for the job. Another way of looking at it is you cannot grow unless you go past your comfort zone, you never stop learning and developing and you have a choice to reframe it as an opportunity, and counter-intuitively as a sign of success. There are lots of people who will want you to succeed so being kind to yourself, recognising you do not need to know everything in the first days, weeks or even months and building relationships with others, including your own staff, many of whom have years of experience, can make all the difference in the world.

1.35 ACTION POINTS

- Assess your current role using the questionnaire provided in Appendix 1.1 and identify areas for improvement.
- Clarify your objectives with your manager within 3 months of starting your job and review them regularly.
- Explore the option of undertaking a clinical leadership or management course, if you have not already done so.
- Make sure there are specific written guidelines that outline the steps you and your staff should follow in the event of a shift being short staffed.
- 'Act up' for your manager to cover annual leave, as a learning opportunity.
- Be specific with others about what your role is and is not.
- Ensure there is an induction/information package for all newcomers to your ward, including doctors.
- Allocate the equivalent of 1 day per week to deal with the administration/paperwork.
- Reduce your patient caseload, see every patient each day and make yourself available at visiting times.

APPENDIX 1.1 QUESTIONNAIRE TO HELP IDENTIFY DEVELOPMENT NEEDS FOR WARD MANAGERS

Leadership Skills

- Does your team have a vision/goal of where you all want to be in a year's time?
- Do you have set objectives/actions that you have identified together to achieve that vision?
- Have you been able to change what is not right/working in your ward/department?
- Have you been able to change what is not right/working in your organisation?
- Have you had discussions with any of the board directors or general managers within the past 3 months about any issues in your ward/department?

- Are you actively involved in any trust-wide initiatives?
- Have you evaluated whether any recent changes in trust strategy could result in harm to your patients?
- Does your ward/department have a high profile within the trust because of high standards and/or quality indicators?

Education

- Are your staff fully trained and developed in all aspects of their work?
- Are you able to access all the educational resources you need for you and your staff?
- Do you know what percentage of your staffing budget is allocated for study?
- Do you plan your staff study leave a year in advance based on appraisal and keeping within the study leave limits?
- If yes to the above, do you involve your whole team in this planning?
- Are all your staff assessed against set clinical competences on a regular basis?
- Do all your staff have a local mentor/facilitator/coach to guide and support their development?
- Do you meet with your link tutor regularly and maintain close relations with the local university?
- Are all your staff up to date with their mandatory training?
- Are you making full use of the in-house and external development programmes to aid career progression of your staff?

Management of Staff

- Have you had an appraisal/personal development plan agreed within the last year?
- Have all your staff been appraised within the past year?
- Do you know who your human resource advisor is?
- Do you meet with him/her regularly to discuss personnel issues (e.g. sickness/absence, staffing issues, recruitment)?
- Have you received training and development on staff management issues such as recruitment, policies and procedures, risk management, etc.?
- Do you have appropriate development programmes in place for your deputy ward sisters/charge nurses?

Management of Budget

- Do you know what your budget is?
- Do you know what your budget is in terms of PAY and NON-PAY?
- Does your current budget reflect the skill mix required (as identified through a formal skill mix review)?
- Have you had any training and development on managing a budget?

- Do you contribute to the yearly business planning process?
- Do you meet with your finance advisor regularly?
- Are your staff all involved in managing the budget?
- Do you manage your team's annual leave throughout the year so that the ward does not have problems with 'meeting the numbers' in the January to March period?
- Do you have adequate resources for your ward in terms of staff and equipment?
- Do you know what services you have agreed to provide as part of your commissioned contracts?

Maintaining Clinical Standards

- Do you manage to see every patient on your ward every day?
- Are you happy that your staff are delivering care to a high standard every day?
- Would you be able to justify in court the way you allocate workloads and patients?
- Are your staff taking full responsibility for the care of their allocated patients?
- Do you have set standards/guidelines for all specialist procedures on your ward?
- Do you have a system within your ward of regularly reviewing themes from complaints, clinical incidents and local audits?
- Do you have a system of keeping your patients informed about the complaint themes and what you are doing about them?
- Are you confident that all your nurses are skilled enough to question inappropriate medical decisions?
- Do you have a plan of action for each serious incident and complaint within your ward/department?
- Do you have a clinical supervisor to constantly challenge you and enable you to keep up to date professionally?
- Have you and your team made any improvements to care within the past 6 months following patient feedback, results of complaints/incidents, audits or quality indicator monitoring?

Communication

- Do you meet with your team at least once each month?
- Do you open and deal with your email on a daily basis?
- Do you appoint someone to 'act up' in your absence?
- Do you keep your matron fully informed of day-to-day operations and liaise on a regular basis?
- Are you fully aware of your responsibilities regarding the Freedom of Information Act and Data Protection Act?
- Does every member of your team have full access to a computer for email, intranet and appropriate research to carry out their role effectively?

- Do you keep yourself and your team fully up to date about what is going on in the rest of your organisation?
- Do you ensure that your voice is heard at the corporate level?
- Do you regularly get staff to shadow you?

Management of Self

- Are you able to be a role model for your staff by working 37.5 h per week, taking your meal/coffee breaks and still being effective?
- Do you plan your work at least a week in advance rather than just getting through everyday crises?
- Do you have a mentor who provides support as well as challenges you in your professional role?

Please note: This questionnaire is designed simply as an aid to stimulate thoughts and is not meant to be prescriptive or an exhaustive list of tasks that should be undertaken. You may find it helpful to identify those sections where there are mostly 'no' answers and think about what you can do to improve your skills in these areas.

REFERENCES

Barnett v. Kensington & Chelsea Hospital Management Committee, 1969. 1 QB 428.

Boahmah, S.A., Spence Laschinger, H.K., Wong, C., Clarke, S., 2018. Effect of transformational leadership on job satisfaction and patient safety outcomes. Nursing Outlook 66 (2), 180–189.

Bolam v. Friern Hospital Management Committee, 1957. 1WLR 582.

Department of Health, 2000. No Secrets: Guidance on Developing and Implementing Multi-Agency Policies and Procedures to Protect Vulnerable Adults from Abuse. Department of Health, London.

Department of Health, 2002. Code of Conduct for NHS Managers.

Department of Health, 2013. Report of the Mid Staffordshire NHS Foundation Trust Public Inquiry London. The Stationary Office Limited.

Healthcare Commission, 2007. Investigation into Outbreaks of Clostridium Difficile at Maidstone and Tunbridge Wells NHS Trust. Healthcare Commission, London.

Kouzes, J.M., Posner, B.Z., 2017. The Leadership Challenge: How to Make Extraordinary Things Happen in Organisations, sixth ed. John Wiley & Sons, Hoboken, New Jersey.

National Audit Office, 2001. Handling Clinical Negligence Claims in England. National Audit Office, London.

NHS Improvement, 2016. Developing People, Improving Care: A National Framework for Action on Improvement and Leadership Development in NHS-Funded Services. NHSI, London.

NHS Resolution, 2018. Annual Report and Accounts. NHS Resolution, London.

Nursing and Midwifery Council, 2015a. The Code: Professional Standards of Practice and Behavior for Nurses and Midwives.

Nursing and Midwifery Council, 2015b. Raising and Escalating Concerns: Guidance for Nurses and Midwives.

Royal College of Nursing, 2009. Breaking Down Barriers, Driving up Standards: The Role of the Ward Sister and Charge Nurse.

Royal College of Nursing, 2017. Safe and Effective Staffing: The Real Picture. RCN, London.

Royal College of Nursing, 2018. Staffing for Safe and Effective Care: Nursing on the Brink. RCN, London.

Spencer, C., Al-Sadoon, T., Hemmings, L., Jackson, K., Mulligan, P., 2014. The transition from staff nurse to ward leader. Nursing Times 110 (41), 12–14.

Donohue v. Stevenson, 1932. AC 562.

Sun, B.C., Hsia, R.Y., Weiss, R.E., et al., 2013. Emergency department overcrowding on outcomes of admitted patients. Annals of Emergency Medicine 61 (6), 605–611.

Trustees of London Clinic v. Michael Alan Edgar QBD, (19/4/2000, Hidden J). 2001. (LTL).

Chapter 2

Manage Your Time

As mentioned in the previous chapter, putting in long hours at work does not necessarily mean you are being effective or efficient at your job. Invest time in planning, organising, rearranging, sorting and, most important of all, thinking.

This chapter focuses on how to manage your time more effectively and how to achieve a healthy work/life balance in your role.

2.1 DEFINE YOUR WORKLOAD

Nursing workload is influenced by more than direct patient care, and identifying work that is unnecessary, redundant or more appropriate for assignment to other members of the healthcare team is an important part of the ward manager's role.

The benefits of managing your workload more effectively include:

- Achieving your objectives during the day
- Dealing more effectively with urgent issues as they arise
- Ensuring the work you undertake is in line with your key responsibilities and goals
- Having a clearly communicated system of work practices agreed and understood by all
- Having the confidence to delegate work as you have a system for following up actions
- Allowing you to work in an environment that is conducive to productivity and reduced stress

From NHS Institute for Innovation and Improvement, 2008. The Productive Leader: Releasing Time to Lead. NHSIII, London.

Most ward managers are employed to work 150 h per month. It is worth taking some time to check your diary over the previous months and write down all the commitments you currently have in terms of hours per month, as indicated in Table 2.1. The value of this exercise is to accurately identify what you actually spend your time doing, how much time you allocate to current priorities and mandatory work, and help you identify opportunities to make changes and save time. This exercise also allows you to dispassionately look at where your time is spent, and you may wish to share your findings with your peers or manager, especially if they have done the same thing, lest there is anything you may have left out.

TABLE 2.1 Defining Your Workload in Terms of Hours per Month

Description of Task	Total Hours per Month
Meetings List the meetings you attend, including all one-to-one meetings (if weekly, multiply hours by 4, if quarterly divide hours by 3)	
1. For example, monthly ward managers meeting 2 h	2
2. For example, weekly ward team meeting 1 h	4
3.	
4.	
5.	
6.	
7.	
8.	
9.	
10.	
Emails, voicemail and post How many hours do you need per day for this? 30 min – 1 h a.m., 30 min p.m. perhaps? (multiply this by 20 for the monthly figure)	
Investigating and writing responses to complaints (allow an average of 10 h work per complaint)	
Staffing issues (include appraisals, recruitment, etc.)	
Compiling the monthly roster	
Risk management and governance issues (average time spent on serious incident investigations, audits, pressure sore forms, etc.)	
Teaching (include preparation time)	
Own study/course commitments	
Regular admin/secretarial work (e.g. photocopying)	
Corporate or university work (e.g. 'block' recruitment, interviewing)	
Clinical (time spent on ward as part of clinical shift)	
Other (e.g. current project work)	

TABLE 2.1 Defining Your Workload in Terms of Hours per Month—cont'd

Description of Task	Total Hours per Month
1.	
2.	
3.	
4.	
5.	
Total	

If the total hours add up to more than 150, it means that you do not have enough time to complete what is required. This indicates that in order to fulfil your workload, you are working more than 150 h or not fulfilling your commitments. You may be:

- taking work home,
- staying late regularly,
- not getting things done.

2.2 TAKING WORK HOME OR STAYING LATE REGULARLY?

If you have decided to take work home or stay on late regularly, this is not a sustainable option. You are not looking after yourself as you should be well rested, healthy and have a good work/life balance in order to be effective in your role.

2.3 NOT GETTING THINGS DONE?

If the hours add up to more than 150 and you are not physically working all those hours, it means that some parts of your job are not getting done. You are probably finding that you are continually busy but do not seem to be getting on top of things. Things either get missed or get left undone.

Problems occur when you do not formally prioritise what gets done and what does not. It is often the case that clinical work takes less priority in order to get through the administrative work. If you need to spend less time clinically, then plan it. Do not allow administrative work and meetings to take over and leave you feeling continually busy and overloaded.

2.4 PLAN AND PRIORITISE

Start by removing or reducing tasks in order to bring the total down to 150 h. The first place to start is to list the names of every single meeting you attend, including bed meetings, finance, HR, line manager, quality, etc. on a sticky note. Put the names on the top, on the bottom left-hand corner write the frequency and on the bottom right-hand corner write the length of the meeting.

Do you really need to attend all those meetings? Choose the ones that are essential for the welfare of your patients and staff at a minimum. Create a meeting matrix from high (e.g. one-to-one meetings with your line manager) to low importance/priority and high frequency (daily egg bed meetings) to low frequency (annual fire training). What does it tell you? Are you surprised at the number of meetings you attend?

Some meetings may not be directly about patients but keep you abreast of what is happening in the wider organisation and give you a profile and networking opportunities. This is where a supportive line manager and/or mentor can help you to determine which meetings matter and which ones can be delegated to another member of staff. For instance, if you have staff members who are interested in quality and audit and want to develop their knowledge in this area, you could delegate them to attend as your representative. Ensure you meet with them subsequently to get updates and identify any support you need to provide. It may be possible to eliminate meetings, especially if they can be merged with another.

It may be possible for some meetings to be reduced in length. When superannuation, sick pay, study leave, national insurance, etc. are included, a midrange Band seven earns approximately £27/h at 2018 rates, so a meeting with 10 Band sevens in the room costs over £270/h. Your time is your most important currency so spend it wisely.

Essential work includes:

- speaking with patients/relatives,
- overseeing the staff roster,
- dealing with complaints,
- dealing with incidents,
- reading and dealing with email each day,
- managing and supporting your staff.

Non-essential work may include:

- some project work,
- some corporate work,
- teaching externally to the ward.

Once you have worked out your commitments in terms of hours per month (using the prompts in Table 2.1), it is advisable to meet with your line manager to assist you in making the decisions required to reduce the non-clinical work if necessary.

The next step is to realistically identify how much time you have left to devote to clinical work. It may only be 70–80h per month. If that is the case, plan to split it into specific blocks of clinical time. This could be something like four half shifts per week or whatever works best for you and your unit. Devote that whole time to clinical work without going off to a meeting or into the office halfway through. Avoid interrupting your clinical shift to go off to meetings or into the office to catch up on paperwork.

2.5 CREATING A CALMER, MORE ORGANISED WORK ENVIRONMENT

As well as making things easier to find and save you time and energy, having a well-organised workplace is beneficial to everyone and it demonstrates

- Control
- Professionalism
- Leadership
- Self-discipline

A way to organise your office – and the ward environment – is to apply principles from Toyota's Lean Thinking and in particular a tool called 5S, which is a series of steps and procedures to help you decide what should be kept, where it should be kept and how it should be stored. It is also an excellent way to engage staff and to achieve multidisciplinary input. 5S stands for:

Sort – Get rid of non-essential items and make sure the most frequently used items are close by.

Ask yourself the following questions:

Is it needed?
How many are needed?
Where should it be located?

With every item, you will need to ask yourself these questions

Do I need it?
When did I last use it?
Will anybody else have it, such as the originator of the document?
Could anybody else benefit from it?

As you go through each item separate them into the following groups:

1. Must stay
2. Cannot decide
3. Remove/definitely go

Set in order – Agree on a place for everything and keep everything in its place. It should take no longer than 30s to locate any items.

Ask Yourself These Questions

How long does it take to get things?
How do they find their way back to the area?
How do people remember where things belong?
Where should it be located?

Space for filing should be kept to a minimum as the more storage you have, the greater the temptation to fill it. Ideally, items you access regularly should be reachable from your desk area.

Shine – Keep things clean so you can tell when problems occur. The key point of shine is that maintaining cleanliness should be part of the daily work, not an occasional activity initiated when things get out of hand or too messy. It is important to ensure only the furniture that is necessary is kept, and rubbish bins are a blend of ordinary waste, confidential waste and recycling.

Your office is your embassy and projects the kind of manager you are. If it is really untidy, it will inevitably reflect badly on you as both a manager and leader.

Standardise – Have agreed, consistent processes and 'standard work' for housekeeping and organisation, inclusive of processes. Write down your agreed standards and ensure they are visible to others. Agree who will do what on an ongoing basis, including what will happen during planned or unplanned absences.

Sustain – The final step is to ensure that this is more than just a cleanup and you are driving continuous improvements in your own processes (Dolan and Hawes, 2010). This will include undertaking audits to monitor your own compliance and that of your team as necessary. For instance, standardised operational standards could include:

- Work in progress files are kept updated weekly
- If emails do have to be printed, they are stored in work in progress and destroyed after use
- All personal work notebooks are dated
- Daily/weekly information for the line manager is kept in the labelled in tray

2.6 KEEP EVERYTHING YOU NEED TO DO ON ONE LIST

Write everything down on your list, such as phone calls you need to make, messages to get back to people, reports to be written, project work, etc. All papers associated with your list should be filed away on your computer or in the filing cabinet. The list can run into three or four sheets of A4 paper as long as everything is written down in one place. Keeping one list is simple but effective. It serves to greatly reduce your stress and worry by literally taking things off your mind and putting them down on paper. The basic concept is that you can stay on top and in control of all unfinished work, projects, reports and correspondence. You can also prioritise them in the following manner:

1. Urgent and important
2. Not urgent and important
3. Urgent and not important
4. Not urgent and not important

Ideally, work as much as you can work in priority 2 as this will help you feel less rushed and do as few of priority 4 as you can. It is worth periodically checking these with your line manager to ensure your priorities are aligned. It helps if you mark against each priority task approximately how long that task will take. You can see at a glance which tasks will take just a few minutes, such as making a phone call. You can then concentrate on achieving those when you just have an hour or so in the office. Tasks such as reading or writing a report can be left for when you have a longer time slot.

Get into the habit of noting down everything that requires an action and comes to you via post, email, voicemail or phone on your central list of things to do. File emails and associated attachments on your computer if you need to keep them. As noted above, print them out only if absolutely necessary and destroy rather than file them when finished as it is a waste of time and takes up unnecessary space on your desk or in your filing cabinet.

2.7 SET UP AN EFFICIENT FILING SYSTEM

If there are many files in your cabinet left by the previous post holder and you feel you may need to refer to them at some point, then use different types or colour of label for your own files so you can easily distinguish which are your own.

Under Freedom of Information legislation, copies of documents only need to be kept if you are the originator. If you have a copy within your computer files, throw away the hard copy unless you will be referring to it often.

2.8 ENSURE THE OFFICE ENVIRONMENT IS IN GOOD ORDER

Keep your office space neat and tidy with no overflowing papers or post-it notes everywhere. Keep all stationery aids in a drawer, e.g. pens, stapler and paper clips. The only things directly on your desk should be your in tray, computer screen plus keyboard and telephone. It is not always possible, but if you can, keep your printer on a different shelf/desk, preferably within easy reach of where you sit.

The location of your desk is very important. Your computer screen should be facing away from the window. Any glare from the daylight on your screen will cause strain on your eyes and headaches. If space allows, avoid sitting directly across the desk from members of your team as it reinforces hierarchy and is hardly conducive to collegial working. Likewise, for the same reason, keep chair heights approximately similar. Test this by sitting on 'their' side of the desk in a meeting in a lower chair and it will become plain why this matters as you literally find yourself being looked down upon. Plants and photographs serve to make your office a nice place to spend your time but keep them away from your desk. Other personal items such as tea, handbags and umbrellas should be out of sight in a cupboard or drawer. Ensure you have adequate lighting. Order a desk light as it makes your office more comfortable and is better for reading. Keep a store of printer cartridges, as they tend to run out at the most inconvenient moment.

2.9 CONTROL YOUR DIARY

When you are working a clinical shift, you plan what you are going to do after handover, but it often changes due to patient need. As clinicians we are used to continually altering our plans because looking after patients is unpredictable work. However, while there is a need to be flexible, this approach does not work so well when dealing with the administrative side of your role. You cannot afford to spend your day reacting to events and constantly being interrupted. The time when you are not directly involved in patient care should be planned.

2.10 SET YOURSELF TIME LIMITS

Be realistic about what you can and cannot do. Without limits, you end up being overstretched and working longer hours. Allocate a set time for each piece of work. Allow 1 h to do an appraisal, for example, or 2 h to prepare an important presentation. If the task is not finished by the end of the allocated time, set time for the next administration slot or submit the work as it is. It is no good striving for perfection all the time. Ask yourself, 'Will it do?' Aim to do things well enough. Doing them better than necessary is a waste of your valuable time.

2.11 TAKE YOUR BREAKS

Taking proper breaks will ensure you are refreshed and your batteries are recharged during the shift. You may elect to sit with your staff in the tea room as it is where you can often pick up what is going on, as staff are more relaxed. It is also good to get off the unit periodically and meet with other ward managers over lunch as they often act as support networks, sounding boards and safe learning environments for you. Being the nurse manager can lead to a sense of isolation so spending time with peers can be good for a recharge too.

2.12 PENCIL IN YOUR DIARY

Always use a pencil to write anything in your diary. Meetings are frequently cancelled and rearranged at a later date. By using a pencil, you simply rub things out and save the page getting into an incomprehensible mess. Better still, use an electronic diary if you can.

2.13 BOOK AS MUCH ANNUAL LEAVE AS YOU CAN IN ADVANCE

Book as much of your annual leave as you can at the beginning of each financial year. Plan the time off for you and your family and friends. Many have lost annual leave due to poor planning. Something more important will always come up.

In order to keep yourself healthy and keep work in perspective, try to ensure you do not work more than 3 months without an annual leave break. It really is very important to be in control of your own time as well as your work time.

2.14 KEEP UP WITH YOUR EMAILS

Email is the main form of communication in healthcare, so it is important to set aside time at the beginning and/or end of each day rather than saving them up for your 'admin' days. Also, try not to leave the ward every spare moment to catch up with your emails. It is not good time management but is an easy trap to fall into. When you are working clinically, you should concentrate on being there for your staff and patients.

2.15 DELEGATE YOUR EMAILS TO SOMEONE ELSE IN YOUR ABSENCE

When you are on 'days off' or annual leave, delegate your emails to someone else to deal with. This could be your deputy ward manager, one of your staff nurses or even your ward clerk. It keeps your team informed when you are not there. It is a good development opportunity, particularly for junior sisters and charge nurses. Not only will they delete all the junk mail, read and answer the basic ones on your behalf but also they will gain an excellent insight into your role and responsibilities. You must not give out your password, but you can enable certain named staff to have 'proxy access' to your emails. Ask your IT department to help you set this up if you have not already done so.

It is even better practice to set up auto delete on your email when you are on annual leave so you do not come back to a mountain of emails, even if you have delegated them. Too often ward managers spend the first day or two in their office catching up with hundreds of emails rather than being visible for their staff. An example of an out of office message could read: 'Thank you for your email. As I am on leave until [Date] it has been deleted.

In my absence, please email 'Jane Doe' [contact email] or ring ext. '1234' if you have any urgent queries.

For other messages you may wish to resend your email to me after [Date of return]'

In practice, where this approach is adopted, ward managers receive three to four emails after their return from leave rather than hundreds to wade through to find them. Imagine how many millions of hours of time across the health system that could be saved if everyone did this!

2.16 CONFIDENTIALITY

If you are concerned about confidentiality, then perhaps you need to look at how you and your colleagues are using the email service. You should never use your work email account for private or personal emails. As a general rule, all your emails should come as no surprise if another member of your team gains access to them. Remember the golden rule: 'No email is ever confidential so treat emails like a postcard, not a private letter'. Ensure all your team is aware of this. If you need to discuss confidential information, it should be done face-to-face or on the phone and followed up where appropriate in an email so there is an auditable trail of the conversation.

2.17 FILE EMAILS

Do not get into the habit of printing off emails or attached documents. Create various folders on your computer and file them as you would a piece of paper. Folders should be named for easy recall and key colleagues, such as your line manager, Director of Nursing, etc. may have their own correspondence folder. Use the @ sign at the beginning of a folder will bring it to the top of your folder list.

Always use the organisation's shared drive to file emails away. This is the disk that is backed up each day centrally, so if your computer fails in some way, you will not lose all your files. If you are saving your files on your personal computer (i.e. c:/drive), you risk losing them.

2.18 USING EMAILS AS AN ESSENTIAL TIME MANAGEMENT TOOL

Always use email in preference to the phone whenever you can. It saves a lot of time. Nowadays, if you phone, you rarely get the other person and end up leaving a voicemail. They then call you and leave a voicemail and this can go on for quite some time.

Emails are an incredibly efficient way of working. They save much time but it does depend on the user. You should have a system with emails as you would with post. If you open post then leave it in your in tray, it will get forgotten. The same is for emails. If, for example, you get an email reminding you of a report you are supposed to be working on but have not started, do not leave it in your inbox. Place important work in an Actions folder and schedule when you will be working on it and set yourself reminders where there are deadlines.

Add the task within the email to your 'to-do' list, then either delete or file the email. To reduce distractions, silence the notification that sounds every time you receive an email.

- When sending emails have a clear request in the subject line, such as action required (provide a date), for information only (no action or response required),
- response required.

This will help receivers of your emails to determine their response and encourage them to do likewise for emails to you.

2.19 CUT INTERRUPTIONS

It is generally accepted that the ward manager or nurse-in-charge of the shift deals with all the queries and any tasks that are not directly patient related. When you are working clinically, you learn to deal with constant interruptions, but you cannot work like this when managing the paperwork side of your role. So, when you plan time in your weekly diary for office work, you need to arrange cover on the ward. You cannot be in charge on the ward and work in the office at the same time.

2.20 WARD ROUNDS

Undertake a ward round every day, as it is an important part of understanding your staff, their workload and being a point of contact for your medical, allied health and other colleagues. Most ward managers have some way of getting around to speak to all the patients and staff during the shift. This is often incorporated as part of the drug rounds, doctors' rounds, bedside handover or even a round of making beds. Making time to do this every day helps reduce those constant interruptions when you do eventually go into the office. Ward round initiatives like Red2Green, which are about identifying and eliminating wasted time (red days) and enabling decisions that help patients get through the health system without needless delays (green days) may require more hands-on leadership from you, especially in the early days. It is important you are seen to support new approaches to enabling patient time to be valued and your staff will take their cue from your engagement and commitment.

2.21 LET YOUR STAFF KNOW WHAT YOU ARE DOING IN THE OFFICE

Let your staff know that you need uninterrupted time to deal with your administrative work, such as shortlisting candidates for interviews, compiling next month's roster or writing a business case for more equipment. Healthcare professionals often see office work as unimportant compared with direct patient care, so make sure your staff are aware of exactly what you are doing rather than just calling it 'general paperwork'.

If you keep your office door open most of the time, it will create a safe space for people to drop by and enable you to gauge their emotional well-being. There will be times when you will want to get on with things and if someone comes to your door asking 'Have you got a few minutes?' say so: I am just finishing off this business case, would you mind coming back at 2 p.m. when I can give you my full attention?'. Alternatively, you could say 'I can give you 5 minutes now if it is urgent but if you can wait until 2 p.m. I will have more time for you then'. Use your judgement; if someone appears distressed then do what is right in the moment.

Frequently, however, interruptions are because staff have a quick question for which they will know you know the answer. If you find you get the same questions on a regular basis, start recording them and then type up a 'Top 10 Q&As', laminate it and pin it outside your door. You may find it reduces a surprising number of queries. You could also ask staff to write questions too and they could become your next Q&A poster. It may also help putting the Q&As in the tea room too.

2.22 KEEPING ABREAST OF YOUR READING

Reading can be very time-consuming. In addition, keeping clinically up to date involves a lot of time not only reading but also searching for the relevant information. As an industry, healthcare is particularly adept at producing massive documents, many of which you know you should read but struggle to find the time. It is also difficult to know whether the document is important enough to be read or not which is where your manager, peers and colleagues can really help triage what is important and must be known, what is useful and what is in the non-critical basket.

2.23 SCANNING

Scanning helps you to get a feel for the content without reading it through. It saves you a lot of time and energy. With every new document, all you need to do is read:

- the title,
- the introduction or executive summary,
- the subheadings and the first and last sentence of each paragraph or section,
- the conclusion.

Scanning can be applied to any sort of document. Try not to read any document or letter without scanning it first.

2.24 JOURNAL ARTICLES

Do not keep piles of journals because if you do need to refer to a journal article, you can access them online. Add a file labelled 'Current research' on your PC. If you see an article of interest in a journal, save it to your file and read later when you have time or print it off and leave it in the staff coffee room.

2.25 HOSPITAL NEWSLETTER AND INTERNAL BULLETINS

Leave any current information such as the hospital newsletter or internal bulletins on the coffee table in the staff room. Renew them each week. It will help keep your staff up to date as well.

2.26 GETTING THE BEST FROM MEETINGS

Meetings should be used for bringing together the right skills and experiences to be able to make informed decisions and changes. A meeting is not required simply for information giving. There are far more efficient ways of giving information such as email, communication books and the hospital intranet. The purpose of meetings should be to involve staff, not just to inform them.

Few people have training in how to run a meeting. The following steps are important to get the best from meetings that you attend.

2.26.1 Step 1: Ensure the Purpose Has Been Specified

Formal, regular meetings should have terms of reference (see Appendix 2.1). These make it clear what the meetings are for and the way in which they will be run. Sometimes meetings are held when the distribution of a regular email would suffice.

All one-to-one meetings should have a specific purpose. 'To discuss the incident' is not specific enough. You need to have an outcome such as 'To identify what actions need to be taken following the incident'. Ensuring you have a specific objective stops you wasting valuable time discussing issues without achieving anything.

2.26.2 Step 2: Prepare

Notify the person running the meeting in advance if you have an agenda item and send them any supporting papers. Do not wait to raise it at the meeting as 'any other business' (AOB). AOB should be for urgent matters only. Read the minutes or action notes at least one day beforehand. This ensures that you are familiar with what happened last time and remember what you had agreed to do. It also gives you time to prepare your feedback about your actions if required. If you are not sure about any items on the agenda, ring up beforehand and ask. You cannot prepare or contribute if you do not understand what it is about.

Let people know if you cannot make it, will be late or have to leave before the end. It is considered rude to not turn up to a meeting without sending your apologies. Send an appropriate substitute if you can and, if you do, ensure that person is fully conversant with what the meeting is about, why they are there and that they are confident enough to speak up on your behalf.

For one-to-one meetings, send any items you wish to raise by email in advance. This saves time and gives the other person time to prepare too.

2.26.3 Step 3: Know How to Handle a Poorly Chaired Meeting

This can be difficult to do without challenging or criticising the Chair's competence. However, you can help to steer them in the right direction, with questions such as:

- Do you mind if we quickly run through the purpose of the meeting so I can be clear in my mind?
- Can you summarise that last point for us please?
- Last time we had the meeting, we took the current list of delayed discharges as a starting point. Perhaps it might be helpful if we took that approach again?

2.27 CHAIR MEETINGS EFFECTIVELY

The role of the person holding a meeting with a group of people is to act as the 'group facilitator'. This includes:

- enabling everyone to contribute or have their say,
- ensuring the group comes to a decision or sets actions,
- keeping to time,
- utilising the best of the skills and experience in the room.

Before you chair any meeting, make sure you prepare beforehand:

1. *Familiarise yourself* with the agenda and previous minutes before the meeting.
2. *Sort out the room* to enable you to start on time and reduce interruptions, e.g. silence the phone, put a sign up outside the door and arrange the chairs. Book equipment, such as projectors, flip charts, etc. in advance.
3. *Send out the agenda, minutes and any pre-reading materials* to reach individuals at least 48 h before the meeting if it involves people from other areas. This will not only remind them that the meeting is taking place but will also stimulate them to finish (or start!) the actions they agreed to undertake at the last meeting. Put these details up on your staff noticeboard or communication book if the meeting is for members of your team only.
4. *Start the meeting on time.* If someone comes in late, keep going. Acknowledge them with a nod only. Do not start again. If they sit down and ask where you are at, give a brief summary but do not hold everyone up by going through things all over again.
5. *Thank and welcome participants for attending.* Check that everyone has seen the agenda and minutes. Start with an opening statement to focus the meeting and quickly run through the agenda. Introduce any outside speakers and confirm their place on the agenda. Ask for any items under AOB.

6. *Keep the discussion on track.* If you find that people are becoming sidetracked, bring them back by saying something like 'This is a useful discussion, but we need to concentrate on the main issue. We can put that item on the agenda for a future meeting'. Keep your tone neutral and light.

7. *Control interruptions.* Your role is to ensure everyone has the opportunity to contribute. Deal with interruptions quickly or you will lose control of the meeting. Say something like 'One moment please "Ann", let "Lynda" speak first, then we will come back to your point...'.

8. *Observe everyone in the room.* Make sure that all have a chance to speak. Notice and act if someone is trying to speak but keeps being interrupted, or if someone looks bored or not in tune with what is going on. Notice if someone is aggressive, angry or upset. Say things like 'OK, maybe it's time to let someone else speak on this issue ...' or 'What do you think, Wendy?' or 'Simon, you seem to be concerned about this, am I right?'

9. *Deal with conflict* by pointing out what is happening and saying something like 'Ruth, I think you are taking us off track here'. Usually that will nip things in the bud, and it is important others feel safe to comment on the meeting. When you directly level someone's behaviour, be firm but not accusing.

10. *Ensure everything runs to time.* All agendas should be timed. Preferably, the meeting should last an hour. No meeting should go on for more than 2 h at the very most. If a discussion becomes lengthy or starts going round in circles, summarise where there is common agreement, then ask where you want to go from there.

11. *Summarise* the outcome/decision at the end of each agenda item and who agreed to do what. This confirms the message for everyone and makes it easier for the person taking notes.

12. *End the meeting on time.* Thank everyone for coming and their contributions and confirm the time and place of the next meeting.

13. *Produce action notes* within 48 h of the meeting with a named lead and the agreed timescale, either as part of the minutes but highlighted in bold or as a separate action plan with headings 'Decision', 'Action', 'Who By' and 'Date'.

14. *Do not take notes and chair the meeting at the same time.* Always appoint a minute or note taker at the beginning of each meeting if you have no administrative support. Meet with them immediately after the meeting and go through their notes to support them and check for ambiguities.

2.28 LEARN TO LET GO THROUGH DELEGATION

Delegation is not about dumping the job onto someone else. Nobody likes working for someone who gives them all the rotten jobs. Delegation is about giving someone the responsibility and authority to carry out some work for you that is geared towards aiding their personal development.

Do not delegate jobs where failure to deliver would cause immense problems and do not delegate jobs that may be beyond the person's skills and abilities. The basic rules of good delegation are to:

- present the task as an opportunity or challenge,
- ensure the individuals are fully aware of what is required of them – a written brief may be advisable,
- identify areas where they will need support or further training,
- ensure or give the individuals the appropriate authority to carry out what is required to complete the job,
- agree on timescales,
- encourage them to come back to you as questions may arise to ensure they have the best chance of nipping any potential problems in the bud and explain your thinking to avoid ambiguity,
- give feedback to enable them to learn from the process.

Remember that you still take full responsibility for the completion of the job. When you ask someone to do something for you, you are delegating, not abdicating, your responsibility.

2.29 ARE YOU STILL DOING THE JOB YOU WERE PROMOTED FROM?

It is not uncommon for ward managers to find that they are still doing many aspects of their old job in addition to their new responsibilities. Just because you are good at your job of being a clinical nurse does not mean that you should continue to take a patient caseload each shift. You are now in a position in which you oversee patient care rather than actually carrying it out yourself. Your priority has now changed to ensuring your team has the appropriate skills to be able to deliver that same high standard of care.

It is difficult to let go but if you want to develop in your role as ward manager, you cannot do so unless you delegate your old role.

2.30 DELEGATING TO YOUR DEPUTY

A major aspect of your role is to ensure your deputy develops the appropriate skills to be able to replace you at times of annual leave, sickness and when or if you leave your job. As with your staff, do not delegate parts of a project in the form of tasks – delegate the whole project. If you are going to delegate the investigation of a complaint or serious incident, for example, do not ask them just to investigate and report their findings to you. Give them the responsibility and authority to deal with the whole thing, including writing the patient response or incident report. Your role will be to provide support, advice and guidance throughout.

2.31 DELEGATE EFFECTIVELY

When delegating a task, make sure the person understands what is expected of them. Ask them to repeat it to you so you are sure there is no unintentional misunderstanding. Write down the objectives to ensure you agree what needs to be done, the limits, and ensure the other person has full authority and training if required for carrying out the task.

Delegate gradually, without being too daunting. For example, 'Susan, would you like to have the chance to develop your skills in investigating formal complaints? We have had a letter from a patient about a couple of incidents that happened a few weeks ago. I would like you to have a go at leading the investigation. I will go through the process with you and will make sure you have some extra time out to devote to this. You will have the opportunity to learn how to write a formal response too'.

Take a back seat while they are carrying out the work, making sure they know you are happy to support them if needed. If the task has not been completed to the correct standard, it is usually because the person has not fully understood what was required of them. Always give constructive feedback; that is, praise them for things done well and identify areas for further improvement for the future.

2.32 BE PROACTIVE

2.32.1 Underpromise and Overdeliver

A reputation for delivering on time earns you the reputation of being dependable. The only way you can do this is to ensure that you are not over-optimistic when setting deadlines. If you are asked to investigate and report on an incident within 48 h, say you will need 5 days in order to gather the information, then set about getting the report done over the next 2–3 days. If you hand it in on day 3, people will be impressed, whereas if you had agreed to try and do it within 48 h and then handed it in on day 3, your work would have been late. Setting a longer deadline date also reduces the pressure when you have any unforeseen setbacks, such a staffing crisis, which means you have to step in to support the shift.

Do the same when promising things to your team. If you say you should hopefully have the roster done by Tuesday, your staff will be expecting it done by then. They will not be happy if you produce the final roster on Thursday. However, if you say you will have it ready after the weekend and then produce it on Thursday, your staff will be under the impression that you are incredibly efficient.

2.32.2 Do Not Put Things Off

Avoid putting tasks off because you believe they will be difficult. They often turn out to be easier than you think. Even if they are not easy, start early and you have the time to spend sorting out the difficulties. You can also renegotiate the deadline if necessary.

Always begin reports early. Write an outline to start you off for reports, complaints responses and incident investigations (see Chapter 12). This will help guide you and stop you worrying about what needs to be done. If you do not do this immediately, you will end up putting it off by finding more important things to do, like welcoming interruptions to your office!

2.32.3 Ask for Help

Ward managers tend to work in isolation and are often expected to get on with things. Remember that you have been trained clinically and all this managerial and paperwork stuff is new to you. It all needs to be learnt through experience. And you cannot learn if you struggle to do everything by yourself. You will pick up bad habits, which can then become normal practice.

If you have been delegated a piece of work to do and do not know where to start, go back to the person who delegated it and ask. If you get stuck halfway through the piece of work, go back and ask again. Next time you do a similar piece of work you will have learnt through previous experience rather than having to struggle all over again.

2.32.4 Keep Your Paperwork Organised

Keeping your paperwork organised will make you feel as if you have more control over your work. Your aim is to complete as much work as possible in your 7.5-h day, then when you go home you have earned the right to relax and do your own thing with your family and friends. The important thing is to have your time away from work for *you*. 'You work to live, not live to work'.

2.32.4.1 Action Points

- Define your workload and liaise with your manager to review it if you find that your commitments add up to more than 150 h per month.
- Organise your office space and write everything you need to do on one 'to-do' list.
- Reprioritise your 'to-do' list each day.
- Book all your annual leave at the start of each year. Try not to leave more than 3 months between each leave break.
- Allocate a set time each day to deal with your emails, ensuring that someone has proxy access to deal with them in your absence.
- When doing office work, ensure that you are not interrupted and keep your staff informed about the work you are doing.
- Do not get bogged down reading documents in detail. Scan or speed-read them.
- Cut out all unnecessary meetings that do not benefit you, the team or your patients.
- When delegating work, ensure it is always a learning opportunity. Make sure your team does the same.
- Ensure you underpromise and overdeliver.

APPENDIX 2.1 EXAMPLE OF TERMS OF REFERENCE FOR A MEETING

Delayed Discharge Meetings

Terms of Reference

Purpose

To reduce the number of delayed discharges by making improvements to the overall patient discharge process.

Terms

- Members of the meeting include the following list. Those who cannot attend are required to send an appropriate representative from their area.
- If a member misses more than three meetings in a row, the group will automatically assume that person has resigned.
- Agenda items to be submitted 3 days before the meeting date.
- Meetings will be held on the first and third Monday of each month, starting promptly at 2 p.m. and finishing at 3 p.m.
- Latecomers will be expected to enter quietly and not attempt to interrupt the group by making apologies. The meeting will not be interrupted to update latecomers.
- Anyone who needs to leave early must make this known before the meeting starts.
- The first agenda item is to collate any other business (AOB), which is for emergency or short information items. The only points allowed under AOB will be those that were raised and agreed at the start.
- The second agenda item will always be to check the progress of action points from the previous meeting.

REFERENCES

Dolan, B., Hawes, S., 2010. Lean Thinking and Leadership. NSW Health Nursing and Midwifery Office, Sydney.

NHS Institute for Innovation and Improvement, 2008. The Productive Leader: Releasing Time to Lead. NHSIII, London.

Chapter 3

Create a Positive Working Environment

Creating a positive environment for teams to work in has always been challenging in nursing, but not impossible. Nurses join the profession not for money, but to make a difference in peoples' lives; however, they can become demotivated when external factors impact on their ability to offer the standards of care they desire. Financial constraints, waiting times and staffing issues can all impact on a positive working environment. So, how can we keep a positive environment when the reality is that many of the external factors cannot be resolved quickly?

Helping your team feel they are making a difference is an important element of the ward manager's role. Celebrating successes, and even a simple 'Thank You' at the end of a shift, can change a team's outlook of feeling underappreciated to having a feeling that their hard work has been recognised. When individuals feel empowered, they gain confidence in themselves and their self-esteem grows; this in turn helps improve teamwork, morale and job satisfaction. This eventually cascades down through to every member of the team, almost as a domino effect, resulting in people from cleaners to senior nurses, allied health and medical colleagues feeling appreciated and part of a tight-knit team. Much of the research shows that increasing people's self-worth and confidence at work in achieving things is a great motivator.

Many teams are now under constant unprecedented stress, so, how do we manage to keep their morale up and reduce the effects of burnout? Small and simple changes can have the biggest impact, and the best person to start these small changes is you!

3.1 PLAN AHEAD

Anyone working within the healthcare setting has one common goal. Whether they are the chief executive of the entire organisation or the night porter, everyone is joined together with the same drive, to put the patient at the heart of all we do, and work as a team to achieve this. This gives us a unique advantage over other professions. It means that whoever is in front of you is part of a wider team, and that team all have the same goal. Every person within your team will have a specific skill to help reach your goal. To get the best out of the team, utilise those skills and embrace the diversity of ideas and knowledge in front of you. As a leader, your role is to create a motivating environment to enable your team to flourish; however, there are always challenges when different people and personalities work together. Take a good look at your team now:

1. Are there any problems with lateness and/or sickness?
2. Are any of your staff displaying inappropriate or unprofessional behaviour (e.g. flouting the uniform policy, sloppiness, defensiveness or showing an uncaring attitude)?
3. Are there problems between some members of the team who do not get on?
4. Are problems continually being discussed without any effective action ever taken?
5. Have any cliques formed within the team?

If you answered yes to any of the above questions, it may be a sign that people within your team may need more support. Behaviours like these are common in many working environments; it does not mean that you are failing as a leader or a manager, but they are all things that need to be addressed early to ensure that the most positive working environment is achieved.

Often, the attitudes displayed above have a personal connection to them. For example, if a member of staff is constantly late, in a first instance, ask if everything is ok? Explore and see if there is a reason for them being late. This makes the member of your team feel heard and supported rather than instantly being reprimanded. It may even be helpful to put into perspective the impact of them being late has on the team, such as tired nurses who have worked all day and wanting to go home and seeing their families, being delayed further because of one member of staff being late, and how would they feel if the tables were turned? This does not, however, mean that persistent behaviour like this should be tolerated. Part of our accountability to the organisation and NMC professional code of conduct for nurses is to ensure effective time management, and if the issue does not resolve after reasonable attempts, then it is appropriate to follow a more formal procedure.

Engaging with individuals about these problems may often bring to light deeper problems and taking the time to speak to people individually can be exceptionally beneficial, as there is no pressure from other team members. It is important to ensure your team member knows they are not in trouble, and you simply want to have a deeper understanding of the challenges they are facing. This helps to make sure that your team feels supported as an individual and that they have a safe and confidential platform to speak to you. For a productive and united team, making whole team objectives can improve teamwork and morale. It is important to communicate effectively and ensure you have an understanding of the particular strengths of each individual within your team.

3.1.1 Team Objectives

Team objectives are essential within any kind of healthcare setting, from a ward to the community. Why? Because these objectives help to drive and motivate how the team and area work. They offer a benchmark for people to aspire to, as well as giving external visitors an understanding of the priorities of the team in the context of the wider organisational objectives. So, what are your team's aspirations? What does your team want to change or improve on the ward? You probably know what *you* want and where you are heading, but have you any idea what your team want? Have you sat down with them all and asked them?

Some ward managers will say how they share their vision and goals with their team and keep them fully informed. This is a very 'top-down' autocratic approach. A ward or area of work is more than just one person's vision and goals. You cannot run a successful unit or ward without your team, so why would visions and goals be set without them? Everyone's ideas and vision is important, but not always achievable. That is why having an open forum for staff to explain their goals and the reasons behind them, and potentially, how they envision it being implemented is important. There will be many that are similar, and that is when, you, as a leader, help the team to prioritise and categorise the vision and goals. Once the entire team agrees to this, it helps create ownership of the values everyone wants. It is then important to review these and ensure that they are still relevant to your area of practice and they are aligned with the wider organisation's goals, and if they are not, then reopen the discussion.

3.1.2 Develop a Team Action Plan

Once the main objectives have been agreed, the next step as a team is to agree on actions to achieve them.

If, for example, the team's main objective is to get off work on time at the end of each shift, possible actions could include:

- reviewing the handover system to make it shorter, e.g. structured handover sheets;
- ensuring that the culture of 24-h nursing care is embedded, meaning staff can hand over things without fear of negative feedback;
- submitting a business case for an extra member of staff.

Make sure that the meeting is a balance of problem and solution focus. This means that when a problem is discussed, before moving on, people must offer a solution of how to fix the problem. If there is no immediate resolution, you move on and revisit it at the end. By looking at possible solutions, you are focussing your staffs' minds on what they can do, not what they cannot.

Ensure the actions are SMART, i.e. Specific, Measurable, Achievable, Realistic and have a Timetable. The final agreed action plan should then be reviewed regularly with the team together. Some of the objectives can even be incorporated into induction programmers and performance appraisals.

Having a set vision of where you and your team want to be in a year's time is crucial to effective team working. Incorporate regular 90-day goals to help keep you on track. It is an essential but frequently overlooked part of good leadership.

3.1.3 Communicate Effectively

Effective communication is the linchpin of any successful team and organisation. Communication is often underestimated but getting it wrong can have dramatic consequences.

Communicating effectively starts before we even open our mouths to talk. To be able to communicate effectively, we must first understand the barriers to effective communication.

This is by no means a definitive list, but here are some points to be aware of when speaking to anyone:

1. Body Language – Are you portraying an open body language, or a defensive one? If your arms are crossed against your body, you display a defensive stance, and will instantly put the person trying to communicate at unease. A more open body language, leaning in, arms open, etc. helps to make people feel more comfortable.
2. Listening – Leaders need to be good listeners in order to be good communicators. If you are on broadcast mode all the time, it should be no surprise that your team stop listening.
3. Non-Verbal Communication – Often, we can give away how we feel about a subject without even speaking. Rolling of eyes, minimal eye contact, a disagreeing shake of the head can all undermine the person who is trying to put a point across. Instead, change negative communication to positive whilst they are talking. Nod your head so that they can see you are taking in what they said and keep eye contact with them. This does not mean that you are necessarily agreeing with them but shows that you are respectfully taking their points on board.
4. Physical Barriers – Is your office door closed all the time? Does the team feel they cannot come into your office? Take the physical barriers away, keep your office door open the majority of the time so that they know when it is closed, you are not to be disturbed.
5. Not Paying Attention – Nowadays, there are multiple distractions when trying to have a conversation with someone. These can include mobile phones, computers, emails, even the office phone ringing. If someone needs to have a conversation with you, ensure that they have your undivided attention, or at least let them know if you are expecting a disruption, so that they do not feel that you are not seeing their problem as important.

Although it is important to understand barriers to effective communication, it is also important to understand what effective communication looks like.

1. Active Listening – It is important to listen twice as much as we speak, what does this mean? It means that when you are listening to someone, have your entire focus on that. Reflect back on what they are saying, for example, 'you said this, is that right?' Try to avoid interrupting or talking over people and be interested in what the person has to say.

2. Non-Verbal Communication – As much as this can be a barrier, this is also vital in effective communication. Think about the tone of your voice, eye contact and body language; all of these can count towards effective communication.

3. Ask Open-Ended Questions – This not only gives the person you are communicating with a platform to expand on their ideas but also helps to ensure you have a full understanding of what is being communicated.

4. Be Empathetic – It can be daunting to speak to a manager. Remember how you felt when you were them, and how scared they may be feeling. Be empathetic in your approach, and understand if they get flustered, they may be nervous. Help to put them at ease by starting with some small talk or questions that focus on the other person and/or their lives and remind them that you were where they are now once and can remember how scary it can be sometimes. You may feel the same way the person feels when you were a student nurse; however, it is unlikely you will be seen that way by others, and seeing their world through others' lens is an important part of emotional intelligence.

5. Provide Feedback – Whether it positive or constructive, feedback is essential. It helps the person know that you have understood what they have said. Sometimes feedback may not always be positive, but it is important to avoid making it negative. Share your feedback constructively, for example, instead of saying 'you have not prepared for this at all' say, 'next time, it may be worth looking at XYZ to help enhance your point'.

6. Be Clear and Succinct – Avoid the use of technical jargon and acronyms. It is easy to assume that because you work within the same field that people will understand, but that is not always the case. For instance, in healthcare, the abbreviation PD can stand for the following:
   Peritoneal dialysis
   Paget's disease
   Post-partum depression
   Panic disorder
   Personality disorder
   Paralysing dose
   Practice development
   Position description

And that is not all of them! The rule of thumb is be wary of abbreviations, acronyms and shorthand and at the very least say them in full before reverting to the short version, ensuring everyone knows what you are talking about. For instance, on his first placement on a medical ward, one of the authors (Dolan), who is a qualified mental health nurse, was surprised how many patients appeared to have diagnoses of mental illness until it was pointed out that myocardial infarct (MI) in a medical ward was used to signify a patient had a history of MIs. Awkward!

There are many books on effective communication within nursing (e.g. Gault et al., 2017; Bach and Grant, 2015), which give a comprehensive guide to the successes and pitfalls, and are useful to any nurse, not just leaders and managers.

3.1.4 Know Your Team Well

Knowing your team is key to developing a positive working environment and means you can understand their strengths and weaknesses. This gives you a unique opportunity to pair up people with opposing strengths and weaknesses to help develop one another. This not only helps to develop a person's individual weakness but also helps to develop teamwork by using each other as a learning resource. Taking this approach helps your team members see the faith and respect you have for their skills and gives them the opportunity to share them.

This also shows your team that you have confidence in their ability to work together effectively. There will be times when they will need your guidance as a leader to ensure they are getting the best out of one another. It is also important to try and have one-on-one sessions with each member of staff to talk through any learning and development opportunities to develop their strengths and weaknesses.

3.2 FEEDBACK WITH SINCERITY

3.2.1 A Simple Thank You Can Go a Long Way

'Thank you' are two words that can have a massive impact on a team's morale. Whether the shift is a relatively relaxed and calm one, or one that has pushed staff to the limit, a simple thank you can change how staff feel at the end of it. It shows that you appreciate all they have done during the shift and acknowledges their contribution to the care given. It is important, however, to not use a team thank you for individual praise.

If an individual has gone above and beyond what is expected of them, or have had particularly exceptional feedback, it is important to celebrate that with them. With the introduction of revalidation, writing an email or a letter to document their achievements helps to develop their portfolio and also gives them something tangible to celebrate.

3.2.1.1 Be Genuine

People need genuine feedback to know what they are doing well, and which areas need to be improved, and they should not have to wait until their appraisal to find this out. Make it an aim to provide some sort of feedback to each member of your team on a daily basis. For example, if a member of your staff spotted a patient deteriorating and took corrective action, then tell them, 'Well done. I'm impressed with the way you handled that'.

If you give feedback like this, your staff will know what they did well and ensure they do it next time.

3.2.2 Use General Feedback as an Opportunity for Others to Learn

Ensure, wherever possible and appropriate, you give positive feedback in front of others. It not only makes the individual and team feel good but also helps maintain good performance. They are learning what they should be doing themselves in such circumstances. You also need to ensure members of your staff know when they have not done so well. But never criticise! You want to keep your staff motivated. Always remember the golden rule: with any feedback, whether negative or positive, the person receiving it must end up feeling good about themselves.

3.2.2.1 How to Give Constructive Feedback

All nurses are human, which means everyone of us makes mistakes and gets it wrong. Even leaders and managers will often get things wrong. For the majority, this can be a traumatic thing to go through, and can make staff wonder if they are cut out for the job. Constructive feedback is objective, non-judgemental, based on specific observations and encourages discussion as well as provides reassurance and support. As leaders and managers, it is our responsibility to offer constructive feedback, so that we can highlight the mistake, but offer ways to develop and learn from it. It is important to highlight the positives as well as offering constructive feedback, for example, 'Well done. You did well to lay the patient flat immediately and increase the fluids before calling me. Do remember next time to chart the observations, but overall I am impressed with the way you handled the situation'. The person receiving such feedback will make a mental note to chart the observations down in future, and the most important thing is that their self-esteem remains intact. Better still is to ask them what else could they have done to further improve and if they can identify chart observations themselves it will become even more embedded as they will have come up with a solution rather than simply being told the answer.

It is your role as a leader to increase the confidence and self-esteem of each and every member of your team. They will end up a lot more motivated. You know yourself how good you feel when you receive constructive feedback. When giving any type of constructive feedback, make sure that:

1. *You are objective, not subjective.* In other words, stick to the facts and leave out any personal opinions. Saying, for example, 'You don't appear to be prioritising your work as well as you could be'. will be far more effective and less damaging than saying 'Your work is sloppy and unprofessional'.
2. *You listen carefully and seek to enable the person to come to their own conclusion about what they can do to improve.* You can give them information and share ideas, but if you get them to think of the answer, they will be more likely to put this into action.

3.2.3 People Receive Feedback Even If You Do Not Give It

If you do not give regular feedback, your staff will be left to guess what you are thinking. They will note your body language, listen to gossip or look to others less experienced for feedback, which may not be appropriate. Be proactive and make sure all feedback is given frequently and in a positive manner.

3.2.4 Devote Equal Time to Every Member of Your Team

Treat each of your staff fairly and equitably. When you first become a manager, you may notice that your staff fall into one of two groups. The first group are those who are naturally enthusiastic and motivated. They are generally ambitious, love their job and want to get on. Staff who fall into the second group are those who fulfil the basic requirements of their job but are unwilling to take on any additional responsibilities or get involved in any new initiatives.

It is easy to fall into the trap of devoting more time and effort to staff in the first group. These people want to get on, so you naturally feel they deserve more of your attention. If you do this, you run the risk of creating resentment and ultimately you are discriminating against the other members of your team. It is advisable to ensure that all receive an equal share of your time and resources.

3.2.5 Be Involved in All Appraisals

Make sure you are involved in and sign off all performance appraisals for your team. This does not mean you have to do them all. That would not be a good use of your time. You just need to make sure that you are continuously aware of where your staff are heading in terms of career development and where their strengths and weaknesses lie.

The development needs of your staff are paramount. Sending them away on courses is a very small part of their development. Being aware of their needs and strengths will ensure that you are able to build on them on a regular basis during the working shift.

3.3 DO NOT TALK DISAPPROVINGLY OF OTHERS

It does not matter how much someone frustrates, annoys or upsets you, it is important you do not to let your team see this. They will not respect you for talking about others in such a manner, not least as they will come to the view that if this is how you speak of one of their colleagues, or one of your own, what might you be saying about them? Losing the respect of your team will make your job a lot harder than it already is.

3.3.1 Your Manager(s)

It is important to ensure there is no 'us and them' culture when talking about more senior management colleagues. Regardless of what management position you hold within healthcare, the outcome and goals are always the same: ensuring that patients get the best care possible.

To achieve this, it is important that we have differing managers, some of whom are from a clinical background, and some from a non-clinical background. Both parties have different skill sets to bring to the table. There will always be disagreements, and you may even question their motives behind decisions at times; however, it is essential to remember you are working towards a common goal.

As a ward manager, you are often the bridge between the frontline nursing workforce and the senior management teams, including executives. This can sometimes feel like being between a rock and a hard place situation; however, it is also the ideal place to help bridge the metaphorical divide between the various parties as both translate and contextualise strategic decision-making.

If you feel your own line manager is not particularly good at their job, keep that frustration to yourself. This can be a difficult thing to do but speak with people outside of work about your concerns. The informal 'grapevine' in large public organisations means that very little remains confidential for long, and it is important to act as a role model. It cuts both ways, as your manager is likely to become aware you are bad-mouthing them, which makes it even harder to have a mutually constructive relationship. While it does make life easier, it is not essential to like those with whom you work. Going back to the first principles, that the patient is in the centre of the work of the health service, means it is important to have a constructive working relationship with others.

3.3.2 Look for the Positive in Others

Make it your mission to always see the positive in people. If you hear members of your team talking negatively about their colleagues, either:

1. *Turn the conversation around by mentioning the individual's positive aspects.* It usually has the effect of making the negative talker feel guilty and they tend to stop or
2. *Ask them,* 'Have you told x how you feel?' More often than not, they will not have done so, and again it will usually stop the moaning. They will understand that what you are really saying is, 'If you can't tell this person to their face, then it's not very nice to talk about it behind their back, is it?' but in a nice kind of way!

As their leader, you are your team's role model. If you are consistent in your manner and are never seen to moan or talk disapprovingly of others, your team will hopefully take note and follow in your footsteps. We all come to work to be treated with kindness and respect so it is important that starting with you, civility becomes the norm (Porath, 2018).

3.4 ENCOURAGE YOUR STAFF TO TAKE GREATER RESPONSIBILITY

Empowering staff is not as easy as it sounds. You have to be very confident in the skills of your team. It means that you can no longer have full knowledge of what is going on. When you have overall 24-h responsibility for the welfare of the patients on your ward, it is difficult to devolve responsibility to others.

In order to enable individuals to flourish in your team, you have to let them learn from their experiences, including their mistakes. There are still some wards where the nurse-in-charge has a list of things to do for the patients, such as:

- following up the consultant ward round;
- sorting out some delayed discharges;
- ensuring wound swabs/urine samples are taken;
- ensuring pre-operative patients are all prepared for theatre.

This is a very top-down approach. The nurses who have been allocated their patients, either through patient allocation, team nursing or primary nursing, should be responsible for everything to do with their patient on that shift. This is a more productive way of approaching patient care, as it ensures the nurse responsible for the patient is fully aware of plans surrounding their patient. Although they are responsible for their patient, it does not mean that they must do everything by themselves. It is important as a leader to ensure they can delegate tasks if their workload is heavy, including to you if appropriate.

If a patient's discharge needs to be organised, it should be led by the nurse looking after the patient, but it is not a weakness for them to ask you to help, for example, with making a phone call to transport whilst they speak with the pharmacist for discharge medication. The role of the nurse-in-charge is to assist them should they need it. If there are things to be sorted from ward rounds, for example, it is the patient's nurse who should be dealing with these things; your role is to support them in achieving this.

3.4.1 'Nursing Is a 24-H Role'

Nursing has changed drastically, even in the past decade. The job is more complex than it ever has been, and patients' needs are more complex. This means that the role of the nurse is being stretched further and further. The focus of 24-h nursing care, especially within the hospital setting, is paramount to successful patient-centred care.

As a manager and a leader, it is important to look at the allocation of patients to nursing staff. Distribute the workload evenly and fairly, and encourage staff to delegate tasks if and when appropriate, this includes handing over to the following shift; for example, if it is decided that the patient is to be discharged the following day, the day nurse can try and get the majority of the process in action during the day, then ask the night team to continue this so that when it is time to discharge the following day, everything is ready for the following shift to finalise. As a leader, it is your responsibility to embed this culture within your team, and they will follow by example.

3.4.2 Enable Your Staff to Do More for Their Allocated Patients

Having full responsibility for all aspects of the patient's care is the main way that your staff will learn and develop. It is also highly satisfying and motivating to be totally in charge of all care for a group of patients.

The role of the nurse-in-charge should be to support and coordinate the team, not take over or delegate parts of the care. Nurses and support workers who are given full responsibility for a group of patients are far more likely to be satisfied in their work than those who are expected to carry out only the basic nursing tasks for their patients. You have to trust your staff and trust that they will sort out the patient's discharge arrangements, take that urgent wound swab, speak to the relatives, etc. You also have to support them when they make mistakes. The key is to ensure you support them to learn from any mistakes and for you or the nurse-in-charge to be available and help out when needed. Your team is more likely to develop and flourish in such an environment.

3.4.3 Wards Can Be Unnerving Places

Hospitals are unfamiliar environments to most people. Entering a ward can be an unsettling experience. Most wards now have a uniform identifying board so that people understand who is on the ward at any one time. This helps to give patients and relatives an understanding of who is who in the team and inspires confidence. If your ward does not have one, it is something that should be worth considering.

Another amazing addition globally is the widespread use of the 'Hello, My Name Is' initiative, founded by Dr Kate Granger and her husband Chris Pointon: a simple and effective phrase that is not only used between staff and patients, but to other staff members to introduce oneself to patients, relatives and colleagues. This is something that should be adopted by all members of the team, and as a leader and manager, you can push for this practice to be embedded in your care.

Relatives may or may not expect their loved ones to be admitted to hospital, which means nerves are easily frayed and tempers easily lost – this is usually reflective of worry and stress. This can lead to members of your team being exposed to unnecessary abuse or harassment. At no point should this be tolerated; however, it is important that you and your team know how to diffuse difficult situations. If your staff do not feel comfortable to deal with this, encourage them to speak to someone more senior; this may be another nurse or you. Often, the root cause of any upset or stress relatives and loved ones come in to contact with is ineffective communication, and often a simple 'I'm sorry' can, where appropriate, be enough to defuse the situation. The sooner the problem is addressed and dealt with, usually the better the outcome. It is important to use the communication skills you use with your staff with your visitors and patients. Give them a platform to voice their concerns, and actively listen and ask them how they would like their perceived problem to be resolved. If they do not know how they would like it to be resolved, go through options with them, and always advise them to speak with the patient advice and liaison service if they feel they need some more impartial input.

Although the majority of upset can be dealt with at a local level, there are times when relatives' behaviours are not to be tolerated. Any acts of violence and aggression – be it verbal or physical should – not be tolerated. No one comes to work to be harassed in any way. It is important to be empathetic to the situation, but it is also imperative that unacceptable behaviour is not tolerated. If you are ever concerned about anyone's well-being, including the angry party, call security immediately. Ensure that your staff knows how to keep themselves safe in situations, and that lone worker policies are understood. Every hospital has a policy with regard to aggressive and abusive visitors and patients – it is useful to ensure you know where this policy is to help with any complex decision-making. It is also important for staff to know the organisation can press charges against those who perpetrate violence against staff, so documentation is important to assist with these decisions.

3.4.4 First Impressions Always Count

You want the visitors to be happy that your ward is well run and their relative is in safe hands. Even with the advent of primary nursing, team nursing and increased responsibility of staff nurses, relatives still see the ward manager, sister or charge nurse as the one who should know everything. It is advisable to ensure that the nurse-in-charge is available at visiting times. If you ensure they are around to talk to visitors and answer any queries, it will reassure people that they are in control of their work and do not look as if they cannot manage the demands. You need to give the impression and reassurance that the patients on your ward are in safe hands.

Obviously, times have changed and you cannot know everything about every patient on your ward. However, you should know the basic details such as the patient's name and why they are in hospital. Refer them to the appropriate nurse looking after the patient if further information is required. If the member of staff looking after the patient is an inexperienced nurse or healthcare assistant, then stay and support them in giving the information.

3.4.5 Patient Confidentiality

Care plans and evaluations left at the end of patients' beds are inviting for the perusal of visitors. If possible, leave them with the patient at the head of the bed or in their locker. Keep all records behind the reception desk if the patient is not in a position to keep them confidential, such as confused patients or those just returned from surgery.

Use your common sense with regard to the Data Protection Act. There is little wrong with patient name boards at the head or end of the bed. The risk of not having one can be far greater in terms of mixing up patients' treatments. Do not add patient-sensitive information like 'diabetes' for everyone to see, as this may not be the information the patient wishes visitors to know about.

3.5 DEAL WITH TEAM CONFLICT

If staff have arguments or heated discussions in front of patients, take them elsewhere immediately and explain that the behaviour will not be tolerated on the ward. Support your senior staff in doing the same thing. It is important to act as a mediator when situations such as this occur. Take them to a neutral location, away from other staff members, and give them both time to calm down. Explain from the offset that under no circumstances should arguments happen within the clinical area, and that as professionals, they should bring any conflicts into a private area.

Before engaging in a lengthy discussion with those involved, ensure that patients and other staff are safe and that there is enough cover to facilitate them both being off the shop floor. If this is not possible, take it in turn to speak to each individual separately, and organise a time where they can sit together and discuss the event.

Ensure ground rules are maintained; these often include not interrupting one another when discussing their point, not saying anything offensive or derogatory to one another, and also ensuring that passive-aggressive non-verbal communication, such as eye rolling, is not tolerated.

Let them both in turn take the time to explain their version of the situation and advise that it may be prudent for the other to make notes if required.

Once both sides have been discussed, it is your job as a leader to enable the staff members to try and resolve this between the two of them, acting as a mediator and ensuring the conversation is constructive.

Depending on the situation, a conversation can sometimes be enough to resolve the issue, if, however, this is not successful, a more formal approach may be needed.

It is good to ensure you have read policies that relate to this area, such as bullying and harassment in the workplace, grievance process, etc. If you are in any doubt as to how to move forward with this, there is a wealth of resource that you can access, such as speaking with your own line manager for advice or human resources (HR). Each workforce area has their own HR advisor who is specifically trained to deal with this.

It is important to make sure all staff members are involved and asking them to write statements will ensure that information is captured as soon after the incident as possible. If this was an argument where witnesses were present, it would be prudent to collect as much evidence as possible to ensure appropriate action is taken.

It is important to stress that whilst incidents are being investigated, the content should be kept strictly confidential so that all parties have the same level of respect whilst an appropriate resolution is found.

3.5.1 Disciplinary Action

Make sure you know your organisation's disciplinary policy. This outlines what constitutes unacceptable behaviour and the steps to take when such behaviour is displayed (see Chapter 4). Do not threaten disciplinary action as it can only be taken after a formal investigation.

If someone's behaviour is unacceptable under the terms of the disciplinary policy, seek advice from your HR department about instigating a formal investigation. It is advisable to ensure you are familiar with what sorts of behaviour are not acceptable according to your organisation's policy. As the manager, you may have to make decisive action in such situations, and it is best to make sure that you have the appropriate knowledge to do so.

3.5.2 Do Not Allow Disagreements to Get Out of Hand

There are still some wards and departments in which some health professionals within a team do not speak to each other or do not get on. Allowing these situations to continue can have major knock-on effects.

1. It may have a detrimental effect on the rest of the team who may find they are working in an uncomfortable environment.
2. It may lead to mistakes being made if they do not feel as if they are able to ask appropriate questions, or if there is conflict in answers.
3. It can affect the standards of patient care due to a lack of teamwork.

Do not allow it to happen on your ward. If you have a situation like this and feel unable to handle it, get help. Although you are the manager and leader, it is important to stress that you are not the most senior person. You have a wealth of other people who can support you in dealing with this, and they should be utilised.

3.5.3 Bullying or Harassment

If any of your staff are bullying or harassing others, you must also take action as it should not be tolerated under any circumstances since it undermines physical and mental health, frequently resulting in poor work performance.

Bullying and harassment is a form of violence and constitutes a violation of human and legal rights that can lead to criminal prosecution and civil law claims. Employers have a duty of care to provide a safe and healthy working environment for their staff, and this is an implied term of every contract of employment (RCN, 2015). Wright and Khatri (2015) linked bullying behaviours to poor patient outcomes and when nursing staff feel cared for and supported in their organisation, this leads to better patient outcomes. Conversely, where organisations do not support their nursing staff, be that in relation to responding to bullying behaviours or reducing work-related stress, patient outcomes are affected (NIHR, 2012).

If you have a situation where another health professional is behaving aggressively towards your staff, it is your duty to protect your staff member. Consult your bullying and harassment policy and involve HR right from the beginning.

It is usually advisable in the first instance to help and support the individual to deal with the situation themselves. If you take over immediately, it may only serve to reduce their self-esteem even further. To be able to confront someone who is bullying or harassing them with your full support may give the individual a greater sense of satisfaction and self-worth. Effective people management is the most successful counter to bullying and harassment (RCN, 2015).

3.5.4 Not All Confrontation Is Detrimental

Conflict at work is not always a bad thing and maintaining the status quo is not always the best option. Encouraging people to speak up and confront people or situations that may be harmful for the patients should be encouraged. Questioning why you are being asked to do what you are doing is something that should be encouraged within the healthcare setting. It means that staff have a better understanding of what is being asked of them and can clarify any concerns. It should be encouraged and praised.

It is essential that you support your staff asking questions. No question is stupid! If you find you are coming up again resistance to asking questions, this needs to be addressed.

3.6 IMPLEMENT CLINICAL SUPERVISION

3.6.1 Why Have Clinical Supervision?

Nursing care and clinical treatments are continually changing and being updated. Unfortunately, whether or not they have a degree, it does not give nurses skills for life. A lot of nursing skills can only be gained through experience. Skills such as dealing with bereaved relatives, counselling a patient prior to disfiguring surgery or teaching a person newly diagnosed with diabetes how to give their own injections can only be perfected through practice. But they can only be perfected if the nurse has someone more experienced to help them reflect on their current practice.

3.6.2 All Your Staff Should Have Access to Someone More Experienced

In an ideal world, a practice facilitator would be available at all times on the ward to work with individual staff to give advice, guidance and support and ensure that they reflect and learn from their daily work. The next best thing is to ensure each member of your team has access to a more experienced member of staff whom they can learn from. It does not matter what you call it – mentorship, coaching, facilitation or clinical supervision. In essence, all members of your team should have access to a more experienced member of staff regularly to help them reflect and learn from their everyday experiences.

The most obvious and inexpensive way to do this is to ensure that each junior staff nurse is matched up with a more experienced senior staff nurse, *who is not a direct assessor or allocated to do his or her performance appraisal.*

If the junior member thinks that what they are going to say may influence their performance appraisal, they may be reluctant to be open about their practice.

If you operate team nursing, it might be worth considering allocating each junior nurse a more senior nurse from the opposite team. That way at least there will be more chance of the two of them working the same shifts.

3.6.2.1 One-To-One or Group Supervision?

One-to-one clinical supervision is ideal but expensive. If you are allowing an hour per month for each individual member of your staff to have clinical supervision, it can prove to be very costly unless they can find time during the shift to go off somewhere quiet for an hour. It is also not especially realistic if you have chronic staffing shortages. A less expensive way of ensuring your team are learning from their experiences is through facilitated group supervision; in other words, having someone to facilitate a small group of staff to reflect and learn from their experiences together. Even if they discuss just one issue from one member of the group, the whole group are reflecting and learning from their colleague's experience.

3.6.3 Clinical Supervision Courses

Whether you decide on one-to-one or group supervision, you will need to ensure that the senior members of your team have the appropriate facilitation skills to help others to reflect and learn from their practice. Most organisations offer short courses on developing reflective skills or clinical supervision. It is well worth the investment.

As healthcare professionals, your staff have a duty to continually update themselves by reflecting and learning from their experience and that is now the condition of the NMC's revalidation process where staff have to show evidence of their reflection as part of their revalidation portfolio (NMC, 2015). As their manager, you have a duty to provide the right conditions for doing so.

3.7 ACTION POINTS

- Use your next few team meetings or arrange a couple of awaydays to identify your priorities as a team and agree specific team goals to achieve over the coming year.
- Each time a member of staff comes to you with a concern, take time to really listen before giving advice.
- Give specific feedback to each member of staff that works with you on your shift. Do this every shift.
- Consider how your team are allocating patients. Are all staff being given the opportunity to have full responsibility for their patients?
- Put up an information board for visitors at the entrance to the ward or review the one you have to ensure it is clear where to go and who to see.

- Read your local disciplinary policy to ensure you are familiar with what your organisation defines as unacceptable behaviour.
- Find out what courses are available for the senior members of your staff to develop their clinical supervision skills.

REFERENCES

Bach, S., Grant, A., 2015. Communication and Interpersonal Skills in Nursing. Sage, London.

Gault, I., Shapcott, J., Luthi, A., Reid, G., 2017. Communicating in Nursing and Healthcare: A Guide for Compassionate Practice. Sage, London.

National Institute for Health Research, 2012. Exploring the Relationship between Patients' Experiences of Care and the Influence of Staff Motivation Affect and Wellbeing. NIHR, London.

Nursing and Midwifery Council, 2015. How to Revalidate with the NMC: Requirements for Renewing Your Registration. NMC, London.

Porath, C., 2018. Make civility the norm on your team. Harvard Business Review 91 (1-2), 114–121, 146 .

Royal College of Nursing, 2015a. Bullying and Harassment at Work: A Guide for RCN Members. RCN, London.

Royal College of Nursing, 2015b. Bullying and Harassment: Good Practice Guidance for Preventing and Addressing Bullying and Harassment in Health and Social Care Organisations. RCN, London.

Wright, W., Khatri, N., 2015. Bullying among nursing staff: relationship with psychological/behavioural responses of nurses and medical errors. Health Care Management Review 40 (2), 139–147.

Chapter 4

Manage Staff Performance

Managing staff is an important part of the ward manager's role; however, it can be daunting. As described in the previous chapter, it entails supporting them to be informed, involved and empowered in making their own decisions. If you are having problems with the performance of individuals in your team, the first thing to look at is the working environment, not least your own behaviour. This has been covered in Chapter 3 first. Sometimes, even with the right environment and support, you may still come across inappropriate or unacceptable behaviours.

So, what is inappropriate or unacceptable behaviour? In a nutshell, it is the behaviour that disrupts your team, either as a whole or individual member. It can also be the behaviour that is detrimental to patients and their care. This behaviour may also come under more serious categories, such as it being unlawful or unethical behaviours.

Any behaviour that disrupts or upsets others should be acted upon immediately. When behaviours that disrupts or upsets people is allowed to carry on, it becomes more and more difficult to get control over and ultimately can have a lasting damaging effect on the entire team. You owe it to yourself and the rest of the team to deal with any individual behavioural issues swiftly and proactively.

The biggest resource you have available to you when faced with this type of behaviour is knowing how to access and implement relevant policies. Policies can initially feel overwhelming when you first begin to use them; however, they are a huge aid! Using policies often helps to resolve this situation without having to resort to formal procedures; however, if it cannot be resolved informally, there are structured frameworks to guide you through the process.

4.1 GET TO KNOW YOUR HR ADVISOR

As a nurse, your expertise is in caring for patients; you have spent years developing and honing those skills, and it makes you an expert in what you do. This is the same for the human resources workforce; they are experts in their fields, so use them!

Most organizations have large human resource departments to help support managers in ensuring managers can effectively lead their team fairly.

Each area will have an allocated HR advisor who is there to help and guide you, so it makes sense to use this expert advice. Their role is to advise you on the appropriate policies and procedures, which set out the expectations of your organisation and the formal steps you can take if staff behaviour becomes unacceptable.

4.1.1 Let Your Staff Know Who Your HR Advisor Is

Accessing the HR department is not solely the manager's job. Often, staff may have questions, which will need HR advice. Give the team the freedom and support to speak to the HR department themselves. Sometimes, staff may want to speak with HR face to face rather than over the phone, so help to facilitate this wherever possible. It is also helpful to keep a file with HR advice available to staff; this can include contact details and useful policies.

In addition, if your HR advisor is called to help deal with a staff issue while you are on 'days off' or annual leave, your staff will feel more confident in seeking their advice. By keeping your team informed of important HR contacts and policies, you can rest assure that your senior staff will be well supported in your absence.

4.1.2 Learning From Experience

Like you, most HR advisors are also learning from each new experience, but if they do not have experience of a particular problem, they do have direct access to the HR director for advice and guidance, they also gain experience of issues from other departments, such as disciplinary hearings, which they can share with you. Having insight into general HR issues will help you deal with future problems as and when they occur, and you can develop the appropriate wisdom to know when to take risks on behalf of your staff.

4.1.3 Consult the Policy at the Informal Stage

Do not wait to familiarise yourself with the appropriate policy at the point where you feel the issue needs to be dealt with formally as this is often too late. It is advisable to see what is advised at the informal stage as it can frequently help prevent the need to go on to the formal stage.

Most policies set out what to do at the informal stage. If you do not deal with the problem informally as set out in the appropriate policy, you may not be able to proceed to the next stage if the situation does not improve. Your HR advisor is there to support and guide you through all stages when dealing with a staff problem.

4.1.4 Get to Know Each Other's Teams

Often HR advisors have very little clinical exposure and do not have a lot of experience with how wards function on a day-to-day basis. To enhance the relationship between yourself and your team's HR advisor, it may help to invite them to your area, show them around and introduce them to team members.

This helps to impress not only to yourself and the team that your HR advisor is part of your wider team but also to make you HR advisor feel like part of your team and the incredible work you do on a daily basis. When having team meetings, it may help to invite your HR advisor to take part in the discussion; they may be able to bring a new perspective to issues raised.

4.2 WRITE EVERYTHING DOWN

4.2.1 Keep File Notes

After any conversations with team members, it is important to keep a paper trail. This not only covers the classic nursing rule of 'if it's not documented, it didn't happen' but also enables you to reflect on any conversations you may have had with individuals or teams.

Emailing a person after a face-to-face meeting to review the content of the meeting not only gives you a hard copy of a conversation but also helps to show your team member that you have listened to them and understood the content of the conversation. This email/paper trail also gives your team member the opportunity to amend anything they are not happy with. This reduces the risk of anyone disagreeing with something you have said verbally.

If you keep file notes, they will aid you in remembering what was said and when, rather than hazy details. The file notes can be kept either in the person's personal file or a file of your own. They can help months or even years later when an incident involving a member of your staff occurs and you are asked if there have ever been any problems earlier.

4.2.1.1 Do Not Focus on Negative Events

Do not just note negative things that may be useful if an incident occurs subsequently. It is also helpful to make file notes when the member of staff does something positive and is praised for doing so. All the file notes you keep about staff will be a useful aid when you come to doing their appraisal as well as any future references. There is a culture of only sharing negative events within healthcare settings; it is essential to also celebrate success and to acknowledge when team members excel in areas.

4.2.1.2 File Notes Save Time

It can be difficult to fit the writing of file notes into a busy schedule, but once you get into the habit, you will find that they save you time. Make a file note of any meetings you have had either with staff as a group or in one-to-one meetings and remember to share these notes to keep an honest and open dialogue. These notes can prove useful as the basis for the next meeting or review of progress.

4.2.1.3 What You Can and Cannot Include in File Notes

Never write down anything derogatory or subjective, and never write down anything that you cannot justify or substantiate at a later date. All staff have the right to see any documents within their organisation that have their name mentioned (Section 7 of the Data Protection Act, IC 1998). If you keep any notes about anyone, they should never contain anything that you would not want the person to see.

Be open and honest with your staff. Show them the file notes you make, or at least let them know that you will make a note of the conversation you have just had. The file notes enable you to

- carry out better performance appraisals;
- provide an accurate record of events months or even years later if required;
- write informed references for your staff;
- provide information that would help in future decision-making;
- remind you of previous events;
- help you to review progress of certain behaviours or events.

4.2.2 Keep Meeting Notes

When you attend any meetings relevant to your team, keep brief notes and share them with your team. It may also help to invite members of your team to these meetings to help them get a sense of the running of them. It is important to keep minutes of all your own team meetings and then distribute these to the entire team, either via email or within the team's break room. You do not have to keep formal minutes of local team meetings, but they do help to guide further meetings and ensure that people are up to date with the meeting events if they are unable to be present.

4.2.3 Keep a Staff Communication Book and Notice Board

It is a good idea to print off any important emails, new policies or procedures or any written communication that you receive that may affect your staff. Highlight any pertinent bits, particularly on minutes of meetings. It helps them to see quickly which parts of the documents they need to know, rather than being put off by the surrounding jargon.

If you make sure the information is relevant to their day-to-day practice and highlight the relevant parts in any long documents, there is a greater chance that your staff will be motivated to read it.

Many units now support a 'safety huddle' at team handover. This helps to disseminate important information teams need to know before the start of commencing their shift.

4.3 MAKE APPRAISALS WORK

Effective patient care depends on having staff who know what they are doing and why, and are fully knowledgeable, skilled and developed to be able to carry out their work effectively. Appraisal and development planning and review processes should ensure that this occurs throughout the organisation on a regular basis. Effective appraisal and development contributes directly to patient outcomes (NHS Staff Council, 2010).

Many people see appraisals as ways to ensure they get their increment in pay; however, this is the smallest part of the appraisal process. The appraisal is a joint project between the appraiser and appraisee, identifying career paths, celebrating success and giving constructive feedback, so that you provide a platform for every team member to get the most out of their career.

Most organizations offer appraisal training. Utilise this training, not only for you, but also for junior team members so they not only get the best out of their own appraisals but also have the opportunity to undertake appraisals of junior staff themselves.

Appraisals give every member of the team the opportunity to have an open and honest conversation about where they are and where they would like to head.

The deputy ward managers, sisters and charge nurses can do the staff nurse appraisals, and the senior staff nurses can do the appraisals for the healthcare assistants.

The ward manager, however, should see and countersign them all. That way, you can have an idea of what the team's goals are, and how you can help to facilitate this.

4.3.1 How to Approach Appraisals

The purpose of formal appraisals is to enhance a person's development and skills to ensure they are meeting the goals of the team and the organisation. Writing your team member's personal development plan (PDP) is a joint process. It is important to make sure that expectations are managed well and that everyone knows what is realistic.

An individual's PDP should be based on three important documents:

1. Career aspirations
2. Organisational values
3. The Knowledge and Skills Framework (KSF) (if working within the NHS)

4.3.2 Why Some People Do Not Like Appraisals

Some people groan when you mention performance appraisals. This may be either because they have had a previous bad experience or unrealistic goals have been made, making them impossible to reach.

Appraisals are important, but that does not mean they have to be long, difficult processes. They should be a summary that formally acknowledges everything you have said over the past year and sets objectives for the next. If you are giving feedback to all members of staff regularly, then you should need no more than an hour at the very most to carry out a performance appraisal.

4.3.3 Five Steps for a Successful Appraisal

4.3.3.1 Step 1: Self-assessment by Appraisee

A few weeks before the appraisal, ask the appraisee to write down anything they would like to discuss and the objectives they would like to agree at appraisal. Most organisations provide a self-assessment form with questions to help stimulate their thoughts. They may also need to provide some evidence for their KSF requirements. Make sure you let the appraisee know that their notes/provisional evidence will be discussed with their line manager.

4.3.3.2 Step 2: Meet With Your Own Line Manager

Review the self-assessment form with your line manager to ensure the objectives are congruent with the organisation's objectives. They will be able to give advice about where else the appraisee can go for guidance and support in meeting the objectives, and any funding for development can be provisionally agreed.

4.3.3.3 Step 3: Carry Out the Appraisal

Your organisation will provide a specific appraisal form, usually based on the KSF. If possible, ensure you complete the form with the appraisee as part of the review rather than writing it up at a later date. It will save you a lot of time. Another good idea is to encourage the appraisee to write up the agreed objectives and action plan afterwards.

Remember to ensure that the appraisee should be encouraged to talk for as much of the time as possible. It is advisable to start off with a general discussion about how the past year has gone with regard to performance and development, followed by a review of the past year's objectives, followed by an agreement on next year's objectives and a PDP to meet those objectives. Remember that you do not have to focus on formal study or courses for development. Taking on projects with support and feedback can often be just as helpful.

4.3.3.4 Step 4: Agree the Final Appraisal Document

Agree the final document with both the appraisee and your line manager. All three of you should sign it. The same goes for your own staff carrying out appraisals. It is advisable that you agree and sign all those that have been carried out within your team.

4.3.3.5 Step 5: Set a Date for Review

Mark in next year's diary when the next appraisal review is due. You may also want to set a date half way through the year to review the person's progress towards the agreed objectives.

4.3.4 Adapt the Form to the Appraisal, Not the Appraisal to the Form

Try not to focus too much on the actual form. It should be used as a guide. You do not have to fill in all the boxes. Everyone is different and each appraisal will be different. If you focus on just filling in the form, the process can become overly bureaucratic. Your role is to help your staff remove the barriers to achieve success. Focusing on form filling is not being a good role model.

4.4 KNOW HOW TO HANDLE UNACCEPTABLE BEHAVIOUR

If a person's behaviour starts affecting others in the team and reducing morale, it becomes unacceptable and you need to take immediate action.

First, make sure you address the problem behaviour early. Situations such as these are difficult, and you are only human and you will have an emotional reaction to it. As a leader, you cannot allow your feelings to colour your input or behaviour. If you need to take a break before speaking with an individual, do so. This is not a sign of weakness, it is a sign of a responsible leadership, as it ultimately makes sure that you can think and speak objectively and rationally.

Second, arrange to meet with the person as soon as possible. Leaving it will only add to their worry (and yours) and may cause them to become defensive and upset. Generally, it is advised that you try and deal with these things informally at first; however, there can be instances where it is essential to escalate to a formal process immediately. If you are in any doubt, you have resources throughout your organization to help. This can be your HR department, and if it is out of the normal working hours of the HR department, you can escalate through to on call senior management. Remember, you never have to deal with situations on your own; there is always support for you, at any time of the day.

4.4.1 Guidelines for Carrying Out the First Meeting

1. Consider setting an informal agenda. This way, you can ensure that all the topics needing to be covered are set out from the start and can give you guidance and structure to your meeting, without it feeling time limited.

2. Ask them to go through with you their version of the events or incidents in question. Take the time to listen. Try to see their point of view and do not be defensive. Use effective communications skills, such as feeding back what they have said to you, to ensure that you fully understand their perspective.

3. Once you have listened to their version, you can then give your assessment. Refer to facts only, not opinions. Respect their right to disagree with your assessment of the situation.

4. Keep the discussion focused on their behaviours. Do not let them blame personality or another person's actions. An example would be to say, ' ... I hear your point of view with regard to Jane, however, we are here to discuss *your* behaviour'.

5. Summarise the discussion and the agreed actions clearly and succinctly at the end of the meeting. Give the staff member time after the summary to have an open forum to ask any questions they may have with regard to the process going forward. Any situation like this will be stressful to a member of staff, and it is important that they know that they are also being supported.

6. Ensure the meeting is documented. Write up your notes in a factual, concise manner and agree an action plan with a clear timetable. It is then important to ensure this documentation is shared with the person involved, whether this is done via email, or letter.

7. Both you and the employee must sign all documentation. Even if this is just a quick 10-min discussion where the person agrees verbally to improve their behaviour, it should be documented.

8. Always try to end these meetings on a positive note where possible. Offer them the opportunity to speak with you at a later date if they feel they need to do so, but ensure that they are aware that there will be a follow-up meeting to review the matter.

9. It is very important to make sure you follow up the meeting, arrange a date for review of progress. Hopefully the problem will be resolved and you will be able to give positive feedback.

4.4.2 Do Not Allow the Behaviour to Continue

Do not allow the member of staff to continue to practice the unacceptable behaviour in question. If it does continue, despite your efforts, you may have to refer to the appropriate policy guidance. If you do not, the behaviour will only continue or worsen. This can have a detrimental effect not only on staff morale but also on other staff members standards. If not dealt with quickly and efficiently, other team members may also adopt inappropriate behaviour themselves having seen that one person has got away with it. Ensure that staff are aware of the impact that this type of behaviour has not only on other team members but also on patient care.

4.5 HANDLE POOR PERFORMANCE/INCOMPETENCE

4.5.1 What Exactly Is Incompetence?

Before you label a member of your staff as incompetent, first ask yourself, 'How do I know that they are incompetent?' In other words, what criteria are you measuring them up against? Personal opinion is not sufficient. While you may think they are incompetent, another person may not.

Competence should be assessed with reference to the knowledge, skills and aptitudes required for the job you employed someone to do. In other words, you need to have very clear competences or standards against which you can assess their performance. In addition, individuals cannot be deemed incompetent if

- their job description has recently changed;
- new systems or technology has been introduced;
- they are newly appointed.

These are factors beyond their control and it is your job to ensure appropriate support, training and development are given to meet the appropriate competences or standards.

4.5.1.1 Other Causes of Poor Performance

If the person's incompetence is due to ill health, you would need to follow the steps outlined in the sickness/absence policy. Ensure that they are getting the most support available to them, including referring to occupational health (OH), to help support them to be well enough to competently do their job.

If it is due to negligence or general unwillingness to carry out duties properly, then it is usually appropriate to follow the disciplinary procedures for misconduct. It is a good idea to check which policy may be more appropriate for the individual situation. As this is often a rarity, it is important to reach out for help, support and guidance. Using your HR team to help ensure appropriate policies are implemented helps not only to ensure that you are following the correct procedures but also to ensure the member of staff is being managed appropriately and fairly. It is also important that you advise the staff member to contact their union and/or professional body for support as appropriate as may require advice and/or representation.

4.5.2 Procedure for Incompetence

Most competence or capability procedures begin with an informal stage where you are required to meet with the member of staff to clarify their role, what is expected and agree a plan with a timetable to achieve the standards and any training or retraining needs should be established and agreed. Hopefully, with the support of you and your team, the member of staff will improve over the next few weeks/months and no further action will be required.

However, if the problems continue, progression to the formal stage may be indicated. This usually consists of a formal meeting with the member of staff, often with a trade union representative and an HR representative and a further plan with a timetable is then agreed. If it fails again, a further meeting may be agreed with a further plan but this time with a formal, written warning that failure to meet the objectives could lead to dismissal. At this stage, HR will have a much bigger input into this procedure. They will guide and support you throughout this process and may sometimes take the lead in investigations, with you supporting them with supporting evidence.

Throughout the whole process, you need to ensure that you are

- doing everything you can to encourage and facilitate the staff member's improvement, e.g. supernumerary time, 1:1 time;
- appreciating the level of improvement attained throughout the process;
- identifying and dealing with any extenuating circumstances;
- identifying the possibility of moving them to a different ward or department where the skills are better matched to the role.

Capability/competency policies vary between organisations. It is wise to ensure you are familiar with your local policy before taking any steps to deal with a member of staff thought to be incompetent in their role. An informal conversation with HR asking advice on a matter is advisable. This does not mean that HR will be involved unless you request them it, but they can guide you to appropriate policies.

4.6 KNOW WHEN AND HOW TO DISCIPLINE

Never take any action under the disciplinary procedure until you have sought advice from your line manager and HR advisor. It should only be used in extreme cases. Putting a member of your team through the disciplinary process can be very damaging to morale, both for the individual and the rest of the team. If you do have to use a formal disciplinary process, the team member will still require support and guidance. If they do not feel that they would be able to be offered this from you, then it is important to support them to find someone be it from HR or their union/professional body.

4.6.1 Minor Breaches of Conduct

It is better to use a structured meeting or review in cases of minor breaches of conduct or performance. This would constitute an informal discussion, not a disciplinary hearing. It is good practice to make a file note of the conversation and agreed outcomes. Examples of cases that you could deal with on an informal basis include the following:

- failure to carry out reasonable instructions;
- unauthorised absence;

- persistent poor time keeping;
- poor adherence to the uniform policy.

4.6.2 Major Breaches of Conduct

The disciplinary policy is one of the few policies where often the first step is to undertake a formal investigation. This is usually undertaken by someone other than the line manager who is not directly involved in the matter. The formal disciplinary procedure may be used for incidents such as the following:

- physical or verbal assault;
- bullying and harassment of colleagues;
- fraud, e.g. falsely claiming unsocial hours payments;
- negligent behaviour, which seriously threatens the health and safety of others;
- malicious damage;
- theft.

Disciplinary action can only be undertaken once a formal investigation of the incident has been carried out. In some cases, police will also need to be involved. Suspension from duty should only be carried out if the person poses a real threat to either patients or staff. Never suspend a member of staff without consulting your senior manager and HR first, do not be pushed into suspending a member of staff if you feel it is unnecessary.

If the nature of the incident is usually extremely serious, the disciplinary procedure does not consist of a series of meetings like most other policies. It consists of one disciplinary panel, which is brought together to consider the results of the investigation and makes a final decision. The panel usually consists of the general manager and an HR representative, other people present will be the employee, their union representative and, where appropriate, the investigating officer. Witnesses may be required to attend where appropriate. The outcome can be one of the following:

- a verbal warning;
- a first written warning;
- a final written warning;
- a dismissal.

In cases of gross misconduct, the case can also be referred to the Nursing and Midwifery Council (NMC) for further investigation. This may result in the individual's removal from the register. In exceptional cases, the NMC may use an interim order to protect the public from risk and suspend the nurse from practicing while their own investigations of the individual's fitness to practice are ongoing (NMC, 2015, 2017).

4.7 ACTIVELY MANAGE SICK LEAVE

If your team are well motivated, it is less likely that you will have continual sickness/absence problems. If you do, look first at your leadership style and if there is any way that you can improve your teamwork before dealing with the individual. One proxy means of assessing staff well-being is to informally monitor short-term, i.e. ≤3 days sick leave in your unit as it can be a marker of how settled your staff are, because happy units tend to have fewer staff episodes of short-term sick leave. It is also important to note the clear association between healthier organizational culture and workplace culture, and patient outcomes (Braithwaite et al., 2017).

Most sickness/absence policies clearly lay out the steps that your staff should take when they are sick. An employee can self-certify until the seventh calendar day of sickness, and as a manager, you should not ask for medical evidence that they have been ill (RCN, 2018).

The staff member should phone you or the nurse-in-charge and inform you

● when they expect to return to work;
● any work/patient issues that need to be addressed while they are away.

They are usually required to keep in touch at regular intervals and give at least a day's notice before return. You should keep a record of all contacts.

4.7.1 Short-Term Sick Leave

Your job is to make sure that all staff who have been off sick are fit for work on their return and to decide if any special arrangements are needed. This means that you (or your deputy) should see every member of staff on return even if only 1 day's sick was taken; it is important to try and complete this meeting on their first day back after being sick. You could be liable for any incidents if you allow a member of staff to return and look after vulnerable patients when they are clearly not well enough to do so. Likewise, a nurse who does not take sick leave promptly if they have, for instance, flu or norovirus also compromises both patients' safety and colleagues' well-being.

All details should be noted on the person's personnel file. Remember that this is confidential information. As their manager, you are entitled to know about the person's sickness if they have been off for eight or more calendar days, but the rest of the team are not. Keep all staff personal files locked away and do not divulge any information to others. If the individual does not want you to know the nature of their illness, then it is best to ask your OH department to see them to determine on your behalf that they are fit to return to work.

4.7.1.1 Take Action in Cases of Continual Short Episodes of Absence

Organisational policies on sickness may advise a referral to the OH team if staff have more than a certain number of absences over a certain time period; for example, more than three episodes within 6 months. This is usually a formal process, aimed at identifying what support may be necessary to help manage sickness absence levels. OH services will assess the staff member's condition in conjunction with their working environment. They may seek reports and further information from the GP, consultant or other healthcare professional, and will ask for written permission to do this. OH will then make recommendations to you as their manager as to how the sickness should be handled. This may involve reasonable adjustments or redeployment.

OH is not there to force, or put undue pressure on the staff member to return to work before they are well enough to do so. They are there to provide advice about fitness for work (RCN, 2018).

If you refer to the OH team, make sure that you tell them the reason for referral and what you want to know.

1. Do you want them to reassure you that the person is now fit for work?
2. Do you want to know if the sickness leave they are taking is reasonable for their condition?
3. Is the sickness liable to continue?
4. If you consider it excessive, ask what is a reasonable level of sickness for their condition?
5. How you can support them within the workplace to remain as healthy as possible.

Check your organisation's sickness/absence policy. It will outline the steps to take if you have a member of staff who continually takes an unacceptably high amount of sickness despite being declared fit for work by the OH department.

4.7.1.2 What Further Action Can Be Taken?

The procedure usually starts with a meeting to establish the reasons and set targets. If these are not met, the next step is often a formal meeting. This meeting may result in

- a further period of monitoring;
- a further referral to the OH department;
- consideration of a transfer;
- a formal caution for a period of around 6 months.

If attendance does not improve, the next stage may lead to a final formal caution for a period of around 12 months. If the behaviour continues after this stage, many policies will then give you the final option of dismissal after a further review. Once at this stage, your HR advisor will be heavily involved to ensure appropriate processes are followed.

As a ward manager, you do not have the authority to terminate the employment of your staff. This responsibility lies with your own line manager whom you should fully involve at this stage.

4.7.2 Long-Term Sick Leave

Long-term sick leave is dealt with very differently. Long-term sick leave is often defined as leave consisting of 4 weeks or more. There is very little you can do when a member of staff has taken long-term sick leave, but you must make sure that the OH department is fully aware and involved.

Whatever the reason, do not forget about someone who is on long-term sick leave, keep in regular contact. Keep in contact by letter, phone or email, as you are still their manager and therefore should have concern for their welfare.

4.7.2.1 Do Not Allow Long-Term Sick Leave to Affect the Rest of Your Staff

Do not just make do with bank/agency nurses day after day. Can you advertise the post as a secondment for another nurse who wants to gain further experience in your specialty? Can you employ another nurse full time in their place using finances from elsewhere within your directorate? Have you any other vacancies (e.g. healthcare assistant) from which you can transfer the funding and recruit another nurse? You could also see if it is possible for the person to undertake different duties such as administration, while unable to return to clinical duties for a while. Explore all options involving all departments. Do not cope without that member of staff and let the rest of the team suffer.

4.7.2.2 Fit for Return to Work After Long-Term Sick Leave?

Always involve the OH department before allowing a member of staff to return to work following long-term sick leave. A decision needs to be made in conjunction with the returning nurse and the OH department as to the terms of their return. They usually have one of the four options:

1. Return to the same job as before.
2. Return to the same job but with a graduated return, i.e. part time and then full time.
3. Return to the same ward but with modified duties.
4. Return to a different job, on health grounds.

If the OH team determines that the person will be unable to return to work at all, their employment may be terminated on the grounds of incapacity due to ill health. It is important that HR and the individual's union/professional body are involved so they receive ill health retirement or other relevant benefits.

4.7.3 Unauthorised Absence

It is important to take immediate action in any cases of unauthorised absence. If a member of staff does not turn up for work and has made no contact at all, do everything you can to find out where they are. Get someone to physically go around to their home if necessary. Your first major concern is for their welfare. If they are fine, you can deal with it informally depending on the reason. An odd occasion of oversleeping would not warrant formal action, but it would involve a meeting with the person on return.

If you feel they were neglectful, you do have the option of deducting their pay for those days in which they were absent (deducting pay is done either on your electronic roster software or by completing a form that you can get from your HR or finance department). In more persistent or major cases of unauthorised absence, the disciplinary procedure may be instigated.

4.8 ENSURE ALL STAFF HAVE APPROPRIATE TRAINING, DEVELOPMENT AND SUPPORT

All development needs, including courses and training, should be formally identified through the appraisal process. You only have a certain amount of funding for study days and around 1%–2% release time to allocate to your team over the year. Make sure you know exactly what funding you have. You are the budget holder and therefore entitled to have this information. Most areas now have their own practice development or educational teams. It is appropriate to delegate the allocation of study days to them as they may have a more comprehensive idea as to which team members require them.

4.8.1 Induction

Staff induction is the most important teaching package you can have, yet one that is so often neglected. Every new staff member should have the time and opportunity to familiarise themselves with both the organisation and the workings of the ward.

There is no formal requirement as to the length of induction but it would be wise to allocate a minimum of 4–6 weeks at the beginning, aside from the formal organisational induction, during which the new person is supernumerary. This includes members of staff who are transferred internally. If you can, try to include the mandatory training requirements during this 'supernumerary' induction period. It saves a lot of study leave for the rest of the team for the remaining year.

Following this, you would need some sort of local package detailing the clinical competences that need to be met. All newly qualified staff will need to commence a preceptorship programme and be allocated a mentor.

4.8.2 Ward-Based Teaching

Regular ward-based teaching sessions are a must but do not just think up subjects randomly. Use your regular meetings to assess the learning requirements of your staff. Asking staff what teaching sessions they would like is a brilliant way to ensure the learning gaps are understood and acted on as they are brought up. Use your regular reviews of the complaints, incidents and quality indicators to provide information about what your team need. Try to involve the whole team in making such decisions, it is not always just nursing staff that need training; housekeepers and administrative teams are all integral parts of the team and can often be over looked.

4.8.3 Learning From Experience

Courses and study days are not the only methods of learning. One of the best ways of learning is through experience. However, without the appropriate support and guidance systems in place, staff will not learn as much as they can from their experiences. If you put junior members of staff into a situation with no support, it can have a detrimental effective to their confidence, and they may shy away from the opportunity again.

Your job as the ward manager is to make sure systems are in place so that your staff can gain as much learning from their experience as possible. First, you need to make sure that every member of your team has access to either a preceptor or clinical supervisor. This should be someone who is more experienced than them but does not necessarily have to be more senior. This more experienced person should be able to work with them or at least meet with them regularly to help them reflect and learn from their day-to-day experiences. If you do not have the skills or capacity within your team to offer this support, try and encourage individual staff to take part in-group clinical supervision or an action learning set with other staff of similar grades from other wards.

The NMC (2018) describes seven 'platforms' of proficiencies that specify the knowledge and skills that registered nurses must demonstrate when caring for people across all ages and care settings:

1. Being an accountable professional
2. Promoting health and preventing ill health
3. Assessing needs and planning care
4. Providing and evaluating care
5. Leading and managing nursing care and working in teams
6. Improving safety and quality of care
7. Coordinating care

The confidence and ability to think critically, apply knowledge and skills and provide expert, evidence-based, direct nursing care therefore lies at the centre of all registered nursing practice.

4.8.4 Clinical Practice Facilitators

Many hospitals now have staff in the role of clinical practice facilitators who are based in clinical areas and provide support for students and staff as well as providing a vital link with universities. Some cover several wards and departments so it is a good idea to build up a good relationship with your practice facilitator to ensure that your nursing students have a good placement experience, and therefore will want to return to your ward once qualified. The practice facilitators will also support your staff, particularly with students who may need extra assistance to achieve their learning outcomes.

4.8.5 Link Lecturer

Most wards have a link lecturer from their local university. Work closely with them and identify together how you can best utilise their time. Unless you are proactive and build up a good professional relationship with your link lecturer, you may end up receiving the bare minimum from them. Remember to give something back too. There is no reason why you or your team cannot provide input into work at the university too. The more helpful you are to them, the more helpful they will be in return.

4.9 PROVIDE ADDITIONAL SUPPORT FOR MENTORS

The only nurses who can formally mentor nursing students are those who have successfully completed an accredited mentor preparation programme, have attended an update within the previous year and are subject to triennial reviews where they need evidence to show that they have mentored at least two students over a 3-year period. All sign-off mentors must have had additional preparation, which includes being formally observed signing off students on three separate occasions by a practice teacher or another sign-off mentor. It is important to note that sign-off mentors can only sign off the same nursing degree that they hold – for example, a children's nursing student can only be signed off by a registered children's nurse, not an adult registered nurse.

Your organisation has responsibility for keeping these records, and they are checked regularly through NMC visits; however, it is up to you to ensure the records for your area are up to date. It is imperative that you do so, especially in cases where you have to deal with appeals from any failing students.

4.9.1 Failing Students

The most common reason for failing a student is usually that problems or incompetence has not been dealt with in a timely manner. Often, students are subject to 'failure to fail', which is the allocation of pass grades to nursing students who do not display satisfactory clinical performance (Hughes et al., 2016) who in their literature found five main themes to explain why registered nurses continue to pass students through placements:

1. Failing a student is difficult
2. An emotional experience
3. Confidence is required
4. Unsafe student characteristics
5. University support is required to fail students

Students can often not even realise there is a problem until they are being failed. In many cases, the problems will begin to show early on in the student's placement, and it is vital that you identify and document them early on too, do not wait until the midway assessment. If the student has a problem, the mentor should raise it with the student and explore the reasons for their behaviour or competence problem. If the student is made aware early on, they have time to work on making improvements with the help of your team of staff. If the student is not made aware early on and your team do not support the student to improve their performance (and have evidence to show that they have done so), then the student has full grounds for appeal. It is advisable to seek support with the documentation from the link lecturer, personal tutor or practice facilitator.

Encourage your staff to give regular feedback to students on their progress. They should encourage the student to assess themselves and acknowledge their concerns. It is always easier if students can identify their own problems first rather than be told someone else's point of view. Feedback must always be based on competences (i.e. objective), and students should never be compared with others (i.e. subjective). Remember to ensure that the mentors give feedback to their students on what they do well and not to focus only on the negative aspects.

Written evidence always needs to be provided for failing students, but it must be based on observation. Mentors must demonstrate that they have observed the student for at least 40% of their placement, and sign-off mentors need an additional 1 h per week of protected time with their student. It is your duty to ensure that you facilitate this through effective funding and rostering.

4.9.2 Mentor Meetings

Ensure that mentors are given the time and space to meet with their students regularly without interruptions, to discuss their progress. This extra time will have to be planned for within your budget. Do you have funds within your budget to enable mentors to spend time with the nursing students? If not, you should take steps to ensure that it is added.

The mentors should have some sort of forum where they can discuss issues, reflect on their practice and generate ideas for handling various situations.

4.9.3 Reduce Staff Stress

If your staff are stressed at work, it will only serve to increase your problems, including levels of sickness. Stress in the workplace is a health and safety issue, and 38% of staff in NHS England and 33% of staff in NHS Wales reported suffering from work-related stress and/or being unwell in 2013 (Royal College of Physicians, 2015). Organisations are required by law to look at what the risks are and take sensible measures to tackle them (Health and Safety Executive (HSE), 1999). You have certain responsibilities for the health, safety and welfare of your staff. It is important for you to ensure systems are in place to respond to individual concerns. Guidelines are available to help managers meet their legal duties (HSE, 2011). These guidelines outline standards that should be met. Your staff should be able to say that

- they are able to cope with the demands of their job;
- they have a say about the way they work;
- they receive adequate information from you and their colleagues;
- they are not subject to any unacceptable behaviours at work such as bullying;
- they understand their roles and responsibilities;
- they are engaged frequently when undergoing any organisational change.

Some people are more vulnerable to stress than others, particularly if there are recent changes in their personal circumstances. It is important for all staff to feel supported if they are suffering from stress, ensure they know that you are available to speak with if they are feeling they are not coping, and ensure they are aware of OH advice.

4.9.4 Recognise the Signs

Be alert to changes in a person's mood or behaviour, they may become quiet and withdrawn, bossy and aggressive or irritable. Often, these are out of the ordinary for most staff. Take the time for them to know you can see they are not themselves, and offer them support they feel comfortable with. One obvious sign is increased sickness levels or lateness. Other symptoms often missed are becoming too involved at work, staying behind to make sure things are done or expecting higher and higher standards from self and others.

Look out for the physical symptoms too, which can include frequent coughs and colds, headaches, perpetual tiredness and an inability to smile or join in with any banter. The symptoms of stress vary, and if you do not know a person well, it can be difficult to determine. It is therefore imperative that, as their manager, you make it your business to know all the individuals in your team. You should be familiar with how they think, how they organize themselves and how they work together with the others as a team. A noticeable change in someone's behaviour is the main symptom to be alert to; if you do not know how they behave normally, then spotting the changes will be a lot more difficult. Other members of staff may notice these changes, come to you to raise their concerns and take these concerns on-board – small simple attitude behaviours can often be the start of bigger issues.

4.9.5 Reduce the Pressure

Once you have spotted the symptoms of stress, you need to do something about it. The first step is to find out the cause. The only way to find out is to ask and listen closely to what they have to say.

Some common causes of stress in nursing are as follows:

- feeling overloaded;
- feeling out of one's depth;
- feeling undervalued;
- feeling alone and unsupported;
- short staffing and increased demand on services;
- being uncertain about the future, the role or work environment;
- pressures from home such as childcare or money worries;
- being bullied or harassed.

If any of your staff say they feel overloaded, out of their depth, undervalued or alone, then they need extra support. It is important to ensure that they know they have your full support and that you will put processes into place to help them.

Giving support is more than just spending time listening and giving advice. Support involves taking practical action too. If the problem is work overload or feeling out of depth, try working closely with them for a few shifts, observing how they manage their time and helping them to improve any skills deficit. If the problem is feeling undervalued or a lack of confidence, try increasing feedback (both positive and negative) on their day-to-day performance. Consistent feedback helps by showing them what they do right and what they need to do to improve. It helps individuals to take control of their work and feel that they are making progress.

If members of your staff are stressed due to uncertainty about changes at work, this may indicate that either the changes have not been communicated well or they do not understand and need more clarification. Give them an open platform to make sure they feel their opinions are heard and acted upon.

If someone has pressures at home causing undue stress at work, you may not be able to sort out their home circumstances, but consider what you can do to help at work. Possible solutions may include allowing them a short period of leave or a change in working hours.

If any members of your staff are being bullied or harassed, take action to stop it immediately. Give them some time out from the situation or move staff if necessary. Involve HR straight away for advice and support on the best approach to follow. Never leave a situation like this to solve itself.

4.10 INFORM AND INVOLVE ALL OF YOUR TEAM

If people are given a say about the way they do their work, receive adequate information and support and are fully engaged in any organisational changes, they are more likely to maintain high levels of health, well-being and performance (HSE, 2011). In other words, you will have fewer problems with sickness absence, high staff turnover and poor performance.

Be completely open and honest with your team about everything that is going on. Generally the only information that you need to keep confidential is the personal details of your staff members.

4.10.1 Information From Meetings

When you attend the meetings held by your line manager or nursing director, let your staff know of all decisions that have been made and any information you have gained. Just giving your staff the minutes to read through is generally insufficient. They do not know which bits are important and may not understand or have time to read through the jargon. Highlight the parts that are pertinent to them. Clarify for them what the decisions mean.

4.10.2 Involvement in Making Decisions

Keeping staff informed about everything to do with the ward is essential, but even more important is getting them involved. Be honest. If you are unsure how a future change is going to affect their jobs then say so, but make sure you involve them in the process of finding out.

Try not to make all managerial decisions by yourself, involve your team. If, for example, you involve them in managing your budget and the roster, they will understand the importance of ensuring that everyone books their annual leave in advance and therefore will be more likely to do so.

4.10.3 Business Planning and Recruitment

Involve your team in the business planning process each year and in monitoring how the budget is being spent.

Review your budget statement with your team each month. When a member of staff leaves, review with your team what the role should be and what should be put in the advert. Identify who wants to be involved in the interviews and whether the selection process should involve a presentation. This is a far better way of treating your staff than just informing them that your budget is overspent or you are recruiting another member of staff.

4.10.4 Planning the Team's Study Leave

When deciding each year how to allocate your study leave for the team, involve them in that decision too. List all the courses that staff would like to undertake in the coming year and then add up all the study days these will cost the team. Let them know how many study days you have to allocate over the year (usually around 1%–2% of your budget, see Chapter 6) and decide between you who and what take priority.

Your staff will be far more motivated if they can see the restrictions to which you are working. Understanding why the decision needs to be made leaves them a lot less willing to find someone to blame if they cannot have all the study leave they would like. If you are unable to fund study leave, inform staff on how to look for bursaries or external funding and involve your education team who may be able to identify sources of funding.

4.10.5 Investigating Complaints

Investigating and writing a response to a complainant is an excellent learning experience, not only for the person you delegate the investigation to but also for the whole team. Share the results of the investigation and the difficulties you had during the process. Show them the final response letter and ask if they all agree with what you are saying. This not only gives them an insight into the problem, it keeps them involved. It shows that you truly value your team and their opinions.

4.11 CONSIDER TEAM-BASED SELF-ROSTERING

By having shared goals and an action plan, you are well on the way to ensuring your staff work better together. Getting them to appreciate each others' needs is another hurdle. One way you can do this is through team-based self-rostering. Self-rostering does not mean having everyone writing down when they want to work and whoever gets there last gets the worst shift pattern! It also does not mean having everyone fill in their requests on a draft roster. Self-rostering is about giving your staff the flexibility to cover the shifts in their team in their own way instead of your way. It is, however, important to ensure that patient safety is still maintained with appropriate skill mix.

4.11.1 Self-rostering Is Easier in Small Teams

Do not implement self-rostering for the whole team to do at once. There is no way you can get them all together for a start. There are far too many of them, and you cannot leave the ward without cover. The ideal way to self-roster is within teams.

Many wards nowadays are divided into two or three teams. Give each team their part of the roster and ask them to sort it out among themselves to cover their patients on a 24-h basis. They will soon become more aware of each others' needs and more willing to give and take. They will be more aware about who needs to work with their mentor and who needs time off to take their children to football practice every Thursday evening, for example. They will have to decide among themselves who is more deserving of having certain weekends off. They will have to choose between the one who wants to go to the wedding or the one who wants to go to a concert. Leaving it for your staff to decide among themselves in small teams makes them appreciate each others' needs far better than if the decision was left to you.

If you are restricted to having one senior staff nurse on per shift from either team, it may be easier to get one team to do their part of the roster first, then the next team to devise their part around it. They can swap over next time to make the process fair. It ensures that there is always an appropriate senior member in charge per shift.

4.11.2 Advantages of Self-rostering

There are many advantages to team-based self-rostering. The benefits for staff include the following:

- having more control over their working lives;
- covering for each other to fit in with family care arrangements;
- more control to be at work for individual work commitments, e.g. link nurse meetings or patient case conferences;
- more control in planning team activity.

4.11.3 Set Rosters With Set Lines

Another option of giving staff more autonomy in their shift pattern is to have a master roster. This is where each member of staff has a set line within the roster. You can then give your staff the option of swapping lines or individual shifts between themselves to meet their personal requirements. This is less flexible but could be a good starting point rather than going for complete self-rostering straight away.

4.12 ACTION POINTS

- Engage with HR and ask for informal and formal advice.
- Start keeping brief file notes of day-to-day meetings and phone conversations.
- Set up a communication book/folder for staff if you do not have one already. Consider including a 'safety huddle' at the start of each shift so essential information is not missed.
- Delegate appraisals to staff, ensuring they have the appropriate skills to do so, and make appointments in your diary for those you need to do yourself.
- Read through and familiarise yourself with your sickness/absence policy, competence/capability policy and disciplinary policy.
- Make sure you see every member of staff on return from sick leave and make a brief file note if you do not already do so.

- Set dates for monthly staff meetings to review the budget, complaints, serious incidents, etc., and involve your team in any decisions.
- Set up an induction package for all new staff (include all mandatory sessions for the year) and review ongoing teaching packages with your team.
- Set up a regular meeting for your team of mentors to reflect and discuss issues with mentoring students. This can be facilitated by yourself, the practice facilitator or link lecturer.
- Make sure any members of your staff displaying any signs of stress are managed appropriately.

REFERENCES

Braithwaite, J., Herkes, J., Ludlow, K., et al., 2017. Association between organizational and workplace cultures, and patient outcomes: systematic review. BMJ Open 7, e017708. https://doi.org/10.1136/bmjopen-2017-017708.

Health and Safety Executive, 1999. The Management of Health and Safety at Work Regulations.

Health and Safety Executive, 2011. What Are the Management Standards for Work-related Stress? HSE, Suffolk.

Hughes, L.J., Mitchell, M., Johnston, A.M., 2016. Failure to fail in nursing: a systematic integrative literature review in nursing. Nurse Education in Practice 20, 54–63.

NHS Staff Council, 2010. Appraisals and KSF Made Simple – a Practical Guide.

Nursing and Midwifery Council, 2018. Future Nurse: Standards of Proficiency for Registered Nurses. NMC, London.

Nursing and Midwifery Council, 2017. Interim Orders, Their Purpose and Our Powers to Impose Them. NMC, London.

Nursing and Midwifery Council, 2015. The Code: Professional Standards of Practice and Behavior for Nurses and Midwives. NMC, London.

Royal College of Physicians, 2015. Work and Wellbeing in the NHS: Why Staff Health Matters to Patient Care. RCP, London.

Royal College of Nursing, 2018. Sickness Advice Guides. RCN, London.

Chapter 5

Make Sure Care Is Patient-Centred

Many ward managers will say that the care they provide on their ward is patient-centred, but is it really? Truly patient-centred care means that care revolves around the patient's needs, not the staff's needs or ward routines.

The only way to provide truly patient-centred care is to ensure that there are systems and processes in place to find out what your patients really need and then base your care around those needs. This chapter takes a look at those systems and processes required to maintain a high standard of patient-centred care.

5.1 MAINTAIN YOUR CLINICAL SKILLS

Keeping up to date clinically is essential for the ward manager role. You cannot maintain high standards of care without having a thorough knowledge of your speciality. You need an in-depth knowledge of your subject to be able to act as a role model for others. You may also need to protect the patients from others who are less experienced, including junior doctors and therapists.

Having defined your workload (see Chapter 2), you may find that you can spend only four half-days a week on the ward in a clinical capacity, so you should make the most of this time.

5.1.1 Accessing Up-To-Date Information

Make sure you have full access to appropriate up-to-date textbooks on your speciality. Keep them in your office for you and your staff to refer to when necessary. You can source funding for textbooks through:

- your stationery budget
- ward funds
- one of the hospital charities, e.g. League of Friends

You should have full access to professional journals through the NHS library. The NHS Evidence website is accessible to all: http://www.evidence.nhs.uk. Plus, you should have full access to the following:

- NHS Athens if you work in England: http://www.openathens.net
- Health on the Net in Northern Ireland (honni): http://www.honni.qub.ac.uk

- The Knowledge Network for those in Scotland:
  http://www.knowledge.scot.nhs.uk/home.aspx
- NHS Wales e-Library for Health: http://www.wales.nhs.uk/sitesplus/878.

In addition, you should be regularly accessing all sites which offer evidence-based clinical guidelines such as those produced by the National Institute for Health and Clinical Excellence for England and Wales: http://www.nice.org.uk and the Scottish Intercollegiate Guidelines Network: http://www.sign.ac.uk.

Print off any pertinent articles/relevant research and leave copies on the coffee table in the staff room. It is a simple way of enabling both yourself and your staff to keep up to date.

5.1.2 Clinical Supervision

Having an appropriate clinical supervisor is essential for you to help maintain your professional competence and credibility. Find someone who is more experienced and expert than you. One of the senior consultants (nurse or doctor) linked with your ward is a good option. Another more experienced ward manager or perhaps the link lecturer may be suitable. Meet with them regularly to reflect and learn from your experiences. Regular clinical supervision will enable you to:

- avoid picking up bad habits
- challenge yourself and think more deeply about certain areas of practice
- get advice and support

If you cannot find anyone more experienced than you, then the next best option is to set up a group of people and meet once per month to reflect on practice together (see Chapter 10).

5.2 REVERSE MENTORING

Murphy (2012) describes reverse mentoring as 'an innovative way to encourage learning and facilitate cross-generational relationships. It involves the pairing of a younger, junior employee acting as a mentor to share expertise with an older, senior colleague as mentee. The purpose is knowledge sharing, with the mentee focused on learning from the mentor's updated subject or technological expertise and generational perspective. In addition, there is an emphasis on the leadership development of the mentor'.

It takes a degree of courage on the part of both parties to request and provide reverse mentoring and requires considerable trust. That noted, it is also a powerful way of checking in with how your leadership style is landing with others and gives a strong message of leadership humility.

5.2.1 Learning Through Teaching Others

Invite staff or student nurses to shadow you regularly for a shift. This not only gives them valuable experience but their enquiring minds will help stimulate your thinking and question your practice. Giving regular teaching sessions also keeps you abreast of latest developments in your speciality as you cannot simply regurgitate the same content without ensuring you are up to date yourself. Teaching is a valuable learning experience for the teacher as well as the student. And if you find you are unable to answer any questions, go and find out the answer together. There is a saying 'if the student doesn't learn, it's because the teacher didn't teach'. If you are finding that staff are not learning from you, it may not be them, it could be you so ask for feedback constantly that you are being understood.

5.3 ENSURE THAT ALL PATIENTS HAVE A FULL ASSESSMENT AND CARE PLAN

Care planning is an essential part of patient care, but in times of staffing shortages or increased workload it can become low on the priority list for some. Yet without a specific document outlining the plan of care, important issues are likely to be missed. Care planning provides a guide to all who are involved with the patient's care, including temporary staff.

It is essential that all patients are fully assessed, and the written plan of care should be based on that assessment. This may seem basic, but it is still known for some patients to be discharged without having had a nursing assessment or written plan of care throughout their hospital stay.

Care plans save so much time, particularly if you have to use bank and agency nurses regularly. They ensure handovers are safe and efficient. Staff do not have to keep explaining what needs to be done for the patient if it is written in the care plan. Bank and agency nurses do not have to keep interrupting other staff during the course of their shift to ask questions about their patients' care.

If a patient does not have a care plan, nurses have little defence against allegations of negligence. Legally, it will be assumed that the nursing care was not planned if there is no evidence of a care plan.

5.3.1 Which Model?

Roper, Logan and Tierney's model of nursing still appears to be the most popular method in the United Kingdom as it incorporates all activities of daily living. Orem's self-care deficit model and the Neumann systems model are still in use in some areas. Other models include the Gloucester Patient Profile, which focuses solely on physical aspects of care and is useful in auditing and as a trigger tool (Thompson and Wright, 2003).

It is entirely up to you and your team which model you use; just make sure that you choose one that is relevant to your patients' needs and for a good overview of nursing models in practice, read Barrett et al. (2009). You must have some sort of nursing assessment system in place that identifies the patients' nursing requirements, followed by a written plan of care.

5.3.2 Standardised Care Plans

Standardised care plans save time, but your team can adapt them to an individual patient's needs. Sometimes with standardised care plans, people can get used to seeing the same old thing. As a result, you may find that they tend not to read or refer to them. If you specify to your team that they must write the patients' individual needs on the care plan in addition to the routine predicted needs, it will increase the likelihood of them being read.

Some nurses are under the misconception that writing the patient's name under each problem heading is individualising the standardised care plan. This is unnecessary and serves no useful purpose other than to waste precious time. The patient's name only has to be written once on each sheet of paper.

5.3.3 Accountability

As the ward manager, you are responsible for ensuring the *systems* are in place to ensure that every single patient in your ward receives a full nursing assessment and care plan. The registered nurses in your team are responsible for the *content* of the assessment, care plan and subsequent evaluations. The Nursing and Midwifery Council (NMC) code clearly states for nurses that you must: 'Keep clear and accurate records relevant to your practice' (NMC, 2015a).

Get your team together and use their skills and experience to decide on which model is the most appropriate for assessing and planning care for the type of patients you have on your ward. If they have taken part in choosing which model to use, they are more likely to be willing to use that model in their day-to-day practice.

5.3.4 Care Plans as Teaching Tools

Ensure your staff write clear care plans, with specific and measurable goals and actions. For example, a goal for a post-surgical patient such as 'to prevent a chest infection' is not specific. A goal such as 'to remain free from chest infection as evidenced by $T < 37°C$, WBC between 4 and 11, lungs clear on auscultation and negative sputum culture' is a lot more meaningful. When care plans are used this way, they can also be invaluable teaching tools.

5.3.5 Care Plans as Communication Tools

The ultimate purpose of care plans is to inform everyone in the team of the patients' care needs. Any nurse coming back from 'days off' or annual leave and unfamiliar with the patient should be able to find all the information they need in the care plan. If there is no care plan, they will waste time trying to find out.

To condone the non-use of care plans on your ward equates to allowing poor standards of communication and patient care. Lack of care plans increases the risk of untoward incidents and unintentional neglect. Around 10% of NMC hearings concerning fitness to practice are due to allegations of 'failure to maintain accurate records' (NMC, 2011), which includes the lack of care plans.

5.4 BE CLEAR ABOUT WHAT HEALTHCARE ASSISTANTS CAN AND CANNOT DO

Healthcare assistants (HCAs) are an invaluable adjunct in supporting registered nurses; however, there can be confusion around the nurses' accountability for the actions of HCAs. The NMC code states clearly that it is up to the individual nurse delegating the task to decide in each situation whether the HCA has the appropriate skills and competence (NMC, 2015a):

- You must establish that anyone you delegate to is able to carry out your instructions.
- You must confirm that the outcome of any delegated task meets required standards.
- You must make sure that everyone you are responsible for is supervised and supported.

HCAs are as much a part of the team as registered nurses. Unfortunately, there are some managers who insist on having separate handovers for registered staff, and some that do not include HCAs in the handover process at all. Handovers must include the whole team. The registered nurses and HCAs can then plan the care of their patients together.

5.4.1 Give HCAs Responsibility, Not Tasks

Delegating tasks creates a 'them and us' atmosphere. With the emphasis on achieving competencies for diploma (equivalent to NVQ) levels 2, 3 and 4, HCAs are becoming more highly skilled. Rather than delegate a series of tasks to HCAs, it is more appropriate to delegate a small caseload of patients with supervision. This maximises the use of their skills and abilities by enabling them to carry out the care as prescribed in the care plans. It enables HCAs to use their initiative rather than complete a set of delegated tasks. The registered nurses remain available to assist in areas where the HCAs do not have the competence to carry out a nursing task.

HCAs should also be included in all team and decision-making processes. At the time of writing this book, HCAs are not a regulated profession, although in Scotland they are required to comply with the HCA code of conduct, which is regulated through their employing organisation (NHS Scotland, 2011). Given the current trend towards reducing the number of registered nurses while correspondingly increasing the reliance on HCAs, it is likely that some form of regulation will be introduced across the United Kingdom in the future, even if it is simply a code of conduct that is implemented at organisational level. In the meantime, if the registered nurse has ensured that care is delegated according to the specifications of the NMC code as outlined previously, the HCA is then accountable for the care (RCN, 2008).

5.4.2 HCA Training and Development

It is your role as the ward manager to ensure that HCAs have the appropriate training, are assessed as competent and are confident in their own ability to care for patients and perform certain tasks. You must keep records of all training attended and assessments undertaken and ensure that clear guidelines and protocols are in place. It is also advisable that you are familiar with the assessment, training and competences required for each diploma level (levels 2 and 3 enable HCAs to take responsibility for the care of a group of patients whose care plans have already been written by a registered nurse).

Review the HCA job description regularly and ensure it acknowledges any additional responsibilities. The job description should also clearly state the role boundaries.

5.5 NURSING ASSOCIATES

In 2015, Health Education England's Shape of Caring Review (HEE, 2015) identified a gap in skills and knowledge between HCAs and registered nurses.

Health Education England consulted on the nature and purpose of the new role and the government confirmed that it would be a generic role, meaning that qualified nursing associates would have skills and knowledge across the fields of nursing.

Level 5 has been determined as the academic level appropriate for nursing associates, which typically represents 2 years of higher education.

A nursing associate is a new member of the nursing team who will provide care and support for patients and service users. This role is being used and regulated in England and it is intended to address a skills gap between health and care assistants and registered nurses.

Nursing associate is a stand-alone role in its own right and will also provide a progression route into graduate level nursing.

Nursing associates will be trained to work with people of all ages and in a variety of settings. It is intended that the role will enable registered nurses to focus on more complex clinical duties.

5.6 ELIMINATE LONG HANDOVERS

If handovers are continually taking much more than half an hour, then perhaps you and your team need to revise the way they are carried out. Precious time for patient care is being lost as six people in a 30-min handover is a combined 3 h of staff time. Long handovers cause resentment among those hanging around waiting for a well-earned break or to go home. Standardised communication tools such as ISBAR are increasingly popular (Finnigan et al 2010).

Identity – who is the patient, room/bed number?

Situation – condition/status (stable, febrile, drowsy, disorientated, deteriorating, critical). Post-op or waiting for theatre.

Background – brief but relevant medical history, e.g. diabetes, allergies, resuscitation status, interventions/responses.

Assessment and Action (if applicable) vital signs – including Early Warning Score and pain, blood sugars (if relevant), abnormal laboratory results, mobility, medications, skin, psychosocial, other.

Request/recommendations – pending actions, goals, tests and treatments, daily considerations (pressure sores, fall protocols, etc.), discharge requirements.

The shift handover is a crucial period for maintaining communication and continuity of care.

5.6.1 Office Handovers

5.6.1.1 Advantages

Office handovers can be quick and effective if standardised tools like ISBAR are used. They avoid the risk of being continually interrupted by visitors, other health professionals or the patients themselves. There is also minimal risk of other patients and visitors overhearing confidential details.

5.6.1.2 Disadvantages

The problem with office handovers is that the patient is not involved at all. The handover may not always be based on the plan of care, which stays by the patient's bedside. When shut away in the office, the reporting nurse may become judgemental, giving the next shift's nurses preconceived ideas about the patients they are about to care for. In addition, office handovers used alone can become very lengthy, especially if the nurse who cares for the first few patients then has to go and find the relevant nurse to hand over the next few patients and so on.

5.6.2 Bedside Handovers

5.6.2.1 Advantages

Bedside handovers allow for greater patient involvement. Patients have the opportunity to contribute. The nurse taking over for the next shift can put a face to the name and remember more easily who is who without having to resort to the piece of paper in their pocket. It also negates the need for the nurses to visit all the patients after handover to introduce themselves and familiarise themselves with their care plans.

5.6.2.2 Disadvantages

The problem with bedside handovers is that in some areas they have devolved from a 'bedside' handover to an 'end of bed' handover. This rather impersonal approach is similar to some doctors' rounds where the patient care is discussed between health professionals without the participation of the patient. The only patient involvement is through unavoidable eavesdropping. It can also be difficult to maintain patient confidentiality with 'end of bed' handovers.

5.6.3 Combination Handovers

A combination of office handover based on 'name, age and diagnosis' followed by a bedside handover using the care plans can be the most efficient and effective process of handing over between shifts. The first part in the office should be kept brief. The receiving nurses would then divide up into teams to receive a full handover by the patients' beds, but only for the patients they will be looking after. This keeps the handover focused and relevant. It maintains the advantages of each method and reduces the disadvantages.

Ways of reducing the length of handover include:

- handing out printed versions with the patient's name and bed number to each nurse coming on duty
- using taped handovers
- ensuring the handover is based on the patient's care plan
- nurses to only receive detailed handover for the group of patients they have been allocated to care for
- having a system of allocating nurses to patients to ensure that, as far as possible, the same staff care for the same patients each shift.

There have been some studies and general debate about the effectiveness of non-verbal and taped handovers but beware of using these methods as the only means of handover. A report produced by the Health and Safety Executive (Lardner, 1996) into effective shift handover studied five major disasters (including the Piper Alpha disaster) that were caused by faults in the shift handover system. The report concluded that effective shift handovers should always:

- be conducted face-to-face
- be two-way, with both participants taking joint responsibility for ensuring accurate communication
- use verbal and written means of communication
- be given as much time as necessary to ensure accurate communication

5.6.4 Confidentiality and Bedside Handovers

Make sure that your team maintains confidentiality when handing over their patients by the bedside. The nurses should preferably sit down with the patient and discuss the care plan together. This helps to prevent others overhearing. If the patient has visitors, the handover can be carried out quietly and confidentially between the team elsewhere.

It is advisable not to leave the care plans at the end of the patients' beds for anyone, including visitors, to pick up and read. Leave them *with* the patient at the head of the bed or in their bedside locker. If the patient is confused, or unable to look after their care plan for some other reason such as post-surgery, the care plan should be kept somewhere safe such as by the nurses' station.

In addition, you must have some sort of system for your team to dispose of their handover notes at the end of the shift. Order a confidentiality waste bin or a shredder from your stationery budget and put it somewhere prominent in the staff coffee/changing room.

5.6.5 Delegation of Care

Whatever model of nursing care delivery you use, the overall responsibility for the patient's care should be assigned to registered nurses only. However, apart from giving out medications, HCAs who are trained to diploma (or old NVQ) level 2 or level 3 standard are usually competent to implement most of the care that a nurse can. As long as the patients have clear and up-to-date care plans, there is no reason why HCAs cannot be allocated the care of patients under the supervision of a registered nurse. They can make their own decisions as to what gets done and when. It is much better than being allocated tasks. Resorting to task allocation over long periods of time tends to induce apathy and reduce team morale.

5.6.6 Delegation of Tasks

If you have HCAs who have not attained their diploma (or NVQ equivalent) qualification and the associated competences, task allocation may be the most suitable way of allocating the workload. After all, the registered nurses are ultimately accountable for patient care. However, if you do not give your HCAs the opportunity to develop through the diploma system, you are preventing them from taking on additional responsibilities, resulting in unnecessarily high workloads for your registered nurses.

5.6.7 Task Allocation Is Incompatible With the Nursing Process

Although task allocation can be deemed appropriate in some circumstances (i.e. in times of staffing shortages), it is better to aim for a more patient-centred delivery system. The emphasis on tasks removes the notion of individualised patient care. It is therefore incompatible with the nursing process. This probably explains why in some areas it is considered unimportant for patients to have care plans. If the patients do not have care plans and care is centred on achieving tasks, the bulk of the responsibility lies with one person; the nurse-in-charge. This is not an ideal situation. Working towards a team or 'named nurse' approach (or primary nursing) is a much fairer system for all your staff and a more satisfying way of working.

5.7 WORK TOWARDS THE NAMED NURSE (OR PRIMARY NURSING)

To be able to admit a patient, plan their care and look after them every time you are on duty through to their discharge is a very satisfying experience. People take pride in their work. The named nurse does not necessarily have to care for their own patients during their shift. They can delegate to other nurses or HCAs, who can also care for the patient when they are on 'days off'. The named nurse carries responsibility for writing the care plan and ensuring that long-term goals are met, rather than just the short-term goals during the span of one shift.

5.7.1 Patient Allocation

The main problem with patient allocation is that nobody takes responsibility for the whole patient care package. Who is responsible if a patient's discharge was not planned and implemented effectively during their stay? Who is responsible if a patient's condition deteriorated over 3 days and nothing was done? If nurses care for a group of patients on one shift, then another group on the next shift, they will not only have less responsibility but also less pride in a job done well.

5.7.2 Team Nursing

In theory, team nursing is better than patient allocation. The team leader is the person who takes responsibility for each patient in the team from admission through to discharge. In practice, this does not always happen. Some wards simply split the number of beds into two or three groups and allocate a team of nurses to each area. Each team leader then allocates patients to the team members after handover. It then becomes patient allocation but within smaller teams. However, team nursing can help in areas where there are fewer registered nurses.

5.7.3 Named Nurse/Primary Nursing

In theory, named nursing sounds perfect, but when you are 'running on bank and agency' almost every shift, it is not always feasible. However, each named nurse would have other nurses who care for the patient in their absence. It is something that could be quite difficult to organise on a roster when you do not have your full staffing establishment, but once you do, it can work very well.

5.7.4 The Best Method of Care for Your Ward

A simpler way to ensure nurses take more responsibility is to establish a form of named nursing based on the organisation of care that you already have in place in your ward. You just need to establish a system whereby the nurse who undertakes the initial patient assessment and care plan will be the patient's main nurse throughout their stay. If they are coming up for 'days off', it is up to them to ensure that another nurse will take on that responsibility for the next few days instead. The named nurse does not necessarily have to be allocated the patient to care for on every shift (although it is the ideal option). They just need to be the 'named nurse' responsible for ensuring the patient receives the appropriate care, by regularly reviewing the care plan and delegating as necessary.

Accept that the system will not be perfect and you will not be able to ensure it is fully implemented for every single patient who comes to your ward. Fluctuating staffing levels, increased patient turnover and the continual moving of patients from one ward to another make it extremely difficult to run any model of nursing care delivery effectively. The best you can do is to aim for your patients to be content in the knowledge that there is a specific individual who is responsible for their care from admission to discharge.

5.8 MAKE SURE PATIENTS ARE INFORMED

The NMC code states clearly that: 'act in partnership with those receiving care, helping them to access relevant health and social care, information and support when they need it' (NMC, 2015a). In addition, you should ensure the provision of sufficient details about the care, treatment and support options so that patients can make an informed decision (Care Quality Commission (CQC), 2010). As a manager, there are three good systems you can introduce to keep the patient and their relatives informed (and prevent your staff being continually interrupted for basic information):

1. A 'welcome' information board
2. An information board for comments and suggestions
3. Information sheets and leaflets

5.8.1 A 'Welcome' Information Board

Put up a board near the entrance to your ward to inform new patients and relatives when they first come to be admitted or visit. Some suggestions include:

- a welcome sentence in large print
- directions on where to go and who to report to
- a photograph and information on who the ward manager is and their role
- a photograph and information on who the matron is, their role and contact details
- an explanation about who is who and how to identify staff by their uniforms
- which team or individual staff are looking after which bed numbers (no patient names because of confidentiality)
- the number of staff who are or should be on duty
- key patient safety information such as number of days since the numbers of infections (NHS England, 2017), last patient fall, handwashing audits, etc.
- Contact details of the Patient Advice and Liaison Service (PALS)

- the ward layout, including the bed numbers and where they can find the toilets (including directions for visitors' toilets)
- a sentence asking if there is any further information currently not up on the board which they would like to see

5.8.2 An Information Board for Comments and Suggestions

Comments, feedback and suggestions should be welcomed and a 'You said, We did' section that is updated monthly reassures patients and the public that their voice is being heard and acted upon. Details of the PALS should also be placed here too.

5.8.3 Information Sheets and Leaflets

Ensure you have as much written information as you can readily available for patients. Coming into hospital is such an overwhelming experience for some that they may not take in all that is being said and/or may have questions that they do not want to bother staff about.

First, ensure that there is some sort of leaflet or information sheet for when they arrive onto your ward which explains things like what the different uniforms mean and where to get a cup of tea. Many hospitals provide this information in leaflet form. Second, make sure patients have a leaflet explaining their condition or the investigations or surgery they have come in for. There are many good websites that produce information leaflets, which you can download or adapt for your own area, such as the following:

- http://www.patient.co.uk: This has hundreds of leaflets on health and disease, including tests and investigations.
- http://www.medinfo.co.uk: This site provides information sheets for patients on common conditions and drugs.

5.9 PRODUCING YOUR OWN INFORMATION FOR PATIENTS AND RELATIVES

If you wish to produce your own patient information sheets or leaflets within the NHS, there are specific guidelines which you must adhere to regarding the presentation and the need for the appropriate logo and colour. The NHS brand guidelines give guidance on how to devise written information leaflets and provide templates to help you, including access to a downloadable NHS logo (NHS, 2012).

The main things to remember when writing your information sheets or leaflets are the following:

1. Present all information in at least 12-point font, preferably bigger. Arial font is considered the easiest to read.

2. Try not to use words of more than two syllables.
3. Keep the sentences to no more than 15–20 words long.
4. Make it personal by using 'we' and 'you'.
5. Explain any instructions, e.g. if you tell someone not to drive for 2 weeks after the operation, explain why.
6. A question and answer format tends to be more favoured by patients.
7. Cover only one investigation or condition per leaflet.
8. Encourage your staff to write the patient's name on the information sheet, as it will make them more likely to read it.

Ensure the patient information is endorsed by your organisation. If you do not, you could become personally liable for the information given, particularly with regards to clinical advice. Most organisations have a forms committee which oversees all patient information produced internally. Ensure all clinicians (including the consultants) involved in the specialism have had the opportunity to view and comment on the leaflet/information sheet before submitting it to your organisation's patient information group for ratification.

5.10 PERFORMANCE INDICATORS, AUDITS AND BENCHMARKING

5.10.1 Use Audit Tools Wisely

An audit can be observational (e.g. hand hygiene compliance audit) or of charts/medical records (e.g. medical record documentation audit). Clinical audits identify how close performance is to the agreed standards of care (Clinical Excellence Commission, 2016). Estimate how much time you need to audit, for example, how many hours per month you spend filling in forms showing the numbers of patients with infections, pressure ulcers or having had a fall, and get these hours put into your budget in terms of nurses.

5.10.2 Benchmarking

Clinical practice benchmarking is a quality improvement tool. It facilitates, structures and formalises how best practice is compared, shared and developed. It supports nurses in effectively meeting patients' needs. Involvement in clinical practice benchmarking and the opportunity to share good practice rewards those who are willing to share. It inspires nurses to make changes in practice and reassures everyone that they are doing the best they can to develop and improve the quality of care (RCN, 2017). Clinical benchmarking remains a vital tool to ensure that recommendations in reports, such as the Berwick report (2013), are put into clinical practice.

The advantages of benchmarking are as follows:

- provides a systematic approach to the assessment of practice
- promotes reflective practice

- provides an avenue for change in clinical practice
- ensures pockets of innovative practice are not wasted
- reduces repetition of effort and resources
- reduces fragmentation/geographical variations in care
- provides evidence for additional resources
- facilitates multidisciplinary team building and networking
- provides a forum for open and shared learning
- being practitioner led, and giving a sense of ownership
- accelerates quality improvement
- improves the transition of patients across complex organisational care pathways
- Contributes to the NMC revalidation process (NMC, 2015b) in both reflection and Continuing Professional Development elements

As an example of benchmarking, in 2010, the Care Quality Commission refreshed its *Essence of Care* guidelines and it now comprises 12 aspects of care. These are:

1. Safety
2. Self-care
3. Food and drink
4. Personal hygiene and mouth care
5. Bowel and bladder care
6. Pressure ulcers
7. Respect (including privacy and dignity)
8. Communication
9. Care environment
10. Pain
11. Promoting health and well-being
12. Record-keeping (CQC, 2010)

Essence of Care provides a framework to assess practice and continues to look at driving up the quality of care, ensuring that the fundamentals of care are at the centre of the patient experience. Exploring and using the 'best practice' elements within essence of care can help staff assess their own areas. They can compare and share their practices with other health professionals to look at changing elements within their own departments.

5.11 MANAGE STAFFING SHORTAGES

Nursing is currently, and for the foreseeable future, facing extensive and enduring demands on staff. For the first time in years there are now more nurses and midwives leaving the NMC register than joining. The impact of the EU (Brexit) referendum appears to be driving European Economic Area (EEA) nationals away with an almost 90% fall in the number of EEA trained nurses seeking

NMC registration. UK-trained nurses and midwives are also leaving the register, before retirement (RCN, 2017b).

In the long term, your role is to ensure your staffing levels match the workload through:

- effective rostering (including study and annual leave)
- being fully involved in the business planning process, so that you have the appropriate number of staff required for the workload
- taking extra initiatives to recruit and retain staff
- managing staff sickness

In addition, good quality data (HR, quality and outcomes) is the cornerstone of effective staff planning and review. Staffing decisions cannot be made effectively without good quality data on:

Patient mix (acuity/dependency) and service needs and demands
Current staffing (establishment, staff in post)
Factors impinging on daily staffing levels (e.g. unplanned sickness, vacancies, turnover)
Evidence of the effectiveness of staffing – quality patient outcomes/nurse-sensitive indicators such as pressure injuries, falls, etc.

5.11.1 Tactical Responses to Short Staffing

When a shift is short of staff and/or the workload for that day has increased unexpectedly, some adopt the attitude that the team have no other option but to just cope and get on with it. Good leadership is ensuring that the team spends time at the beginning of the shift making conscious decisions about work that will be left undone as well as planning and prioritising the work that needs to be done. For example, if you have two staff down on an early shift (and there are no bank or agency staff available), the rest of the team should not try to get all the work done and resign to accepting incidents where care is substandard. When your team have exhausted all other avenues of getting staff, they must sit down and prioritise. At times like these, you still have to assert some control over your workload. Get your team to decide together at the beginning of the shift what they absolutely must do to maintain the safety of all patients. Then identify together which aspects of care are essential for safety, e.g. food and fluids, medications, constant observation.

These decisions should be made together, documented and the appropriate line manager informed at the beginning of the shift. Do not allow the decision to remain at ward level. The rest of your organisation must be aware of the pressures that your team are under on that shift at the time. Raising the issue at a meeting afterwards is too late. Document what you have done. This should include:

- the reasons for short staffing (e.g. sickness)
- what steps you have taken to try and get further staffing (e.g. other wards, line manager, bank/agency)

- what your team have prioritised during that shift as essential and non-essential
- other actions (e.g. asked bed manager to hold admissions until next shift, etc.)

An incident form, communication book and/or email to the matron/site manager will suffice as evidence that it has been documented. Keep copies.

You owe it to your staff to enable them to make these decisions in times of acute staffing shortages. Your role as a manager is to provide your staff with 'adequate and achievable demands in relation to the agreed hours of work' (Health and Safety Executive, 2011). You would be failing in your duty as a manager if you were to allow your staff to continue to cope in times of acute staffing shortages without giving them the authority and skills to prioritise the aspects of care that must be left undone in order for all patients to be safe. Ensure they document and inform the appropriate senior managers of their decisions.

5.12 TAKE THE LEAD ON WARD ROUNDS

The main role for nurses taking part in ward rounds is to act as the patient's advocate by:

- ensuring the patient is involved in the discussions
- clarifying anything that the patient does not understand
- contributing to decision-making on the patient's behalf
- communicating any changes or decisions to the rest of the team

Attending ward rounds is much more than about taking notes and passing the information on to the rest of the team. It is about identifying the knowledge base and confidence of team members, providing visible support to members of the multi-disciplinary team (especially juniors) and it gives patients confidence that there is visible nursing leadership on the ward where they are receiving care.

5.13 ENSURE THE PATIENT'S OWN NURSE ATTENDS THE WARD ROUND

Nurses are now responsible for the full care of their patients, which means that they are the best people to attend the ward round. With today's high turnover of patients and increasing patient dependency, the nurse-in-charge cannot be expected to know every detail about every patient on their ward. The role of the nurse-in-charge is therefore to ensure that the nurse who attends the ward round is the patient's own nurse, and only to take over when that nurse is unavailable.

5.13.1 Ensure the Patient Is Involved in Discussions

Some healthcare professionals have a tendency to stand at the end of the bed to discuss the patient's treatment and care without including them. In any other situation, this would be considered quite rude but often the patient is too ill and too vulnerable to do anything about it. The nurse can ensure their patient is included by going to sit with them at the bedside. The rest of the ward round members would then have to turn towards the patient when liaising with the nurse. It is a simple and easy way of ensuring the patient is involved.

5.13.2 Clarify Anything That the Patient Does Not Understand

When anyone starts using medical or technical terms, asking the patient if they understand is not always sufficient. Being surrounded by a group of doctors and other healthcare professionals can be quite overwhelming. In these circumstances, it is difficult for patients to ask the right questions. Your role is to assist their understanding, rather than just checking it. It would be far more useful for the patient if you asked them 'Would you like us to explain what the term X means?' rather than 'Do you understand?'

5.13.3 Contribute to Decision-Making on the Patient's Behalf

Your team spend more time with the patients than other healthcare professionals so are usually more aware of their needs than the rest of those attending the ward round. It is therefore only natural that they should contribute to all the decision-making. Part of your role as ward manager should be to spend time developing the skills and confidence of your staff to enable them to speak up on behalf of the patient. Decisions should only be made with full contribution from all members of the multiprofessional team.

5.14 OBSERVE THE PATIENT'S BODY LANGUAGE

Being in hospital is an inherently stressful experience for many patients and their loved ones so be conscious if your patient is being given too much information as they may not be able to take it all in. As their advocate, it is up to you to recognise the signs. Are they looking nervous? Are they looking away from the person speaking to them? A simple question such as 'Are you alright?' or 'Would you prefer to discuss this part of the treatment at a later time?' should be sufficient for the patient to be able to speak up. 'Patients should be given the sense of freedom to indicate when they do not want any (or more) information: this requires skill and understanding from healthcare professionals' (Kennedy, 2001; recommendation 16).

5.14.1 Information Sharing Post Ward Round

In some wards, the nurse-in-charge attends the ward round then goes round to the patients' allocated nurses and explains what decisions were made about changes in care. This so-called 'handoff' duplicates work and increases the risk of key information not being shared, so it makes a lot more sense for the patient's own nurse to attend the ward round. This nurse would note any changes or decisions in the patient's care plan at the time of the ward round. The information should then be passed to everyone by having a short team brief after the ward round with all the team present.

5.14.2 Use Ward Rounds as a Learning Opportunity

Whenever you can, have a junior member of staff or student to accompany you on the ward round. It enables them to understand that attending a ward round is far more than just taking notes. Have them observe the techniques you use in acting as the patient's advocate. Take time after the ward round to discuss what they have learnt. You can send your staff on any number of communication courses, but you cannot beat learning through observation and experience.

5.14.3 Action Points

- Ensure that you and your staff have full access to relevant and up-to-date clinical information both online and via textbooks and downloaded journal articles.
- Make sure your team are aware that full assessments and care plans are mandatory for all patients admitted to your ward.
- Include HCAs and nurse associates in handovers, decision-making processes and planning care if you do not already do so.
- Review your handover system if it is taking too long.
- Review the system you use for organising patient care if it does not ensure that one registered nurse is responsible for a patient's care from admission through to discharge.
- Put up information boards at the entrance to your ward to welcome all visitors, give appropriate information and invite comments/suggestions.
- Use audits, benchmarking and quality indicators to improve care but do not allow the associated paperwork to take priority over actual patient care.
- Give your staff the skills and authority to prioritise and let go of non-essential tasks in times of acute staffing shortages.
- Develop the skills of your staff in acting as the patient's advocate during ward rounds.

REFERENCES

Barrett, D., Wilson, B., Woollands, A., 2009. Care Planning: A Guide for Nurses. Pearson Education, Harlow.
Care Quality Commission, 2010. Essential Standards of Quality and Safety.
Clinical Excellence Commission, 2016. Clinician's Guide to Quality and Safety. Clinical Excellence Commission, Sydney.

Health Education England, 2015. The Shape of Caring: A Review of the Future Education and Training of Registered Nurses and Care Assistants. HEE, London.

Health and Safety Executive, 2011. The Management Standards for Work-Related Stress.

Kennedy, I., 2001. Learning from Bristol: The Report of the Public Inquiry into Children's Heart Surgery at the Bristol Royal Infirmary. 1984–1995.

Lardner, R., 1996. Effective Shift Handover – a Literature Review. HSE, Suffolk.

Murphy, W.M., 2012. Reverse Mentoring at work: fostering cross-generational learning and developing millennial leaders. Human Resource Management 51 (4), 549–574.

NHS England, 2017. Next Steps on the Five Year Forward View. NHS England, London.

NHS, 2012. The NHS Brand Guidelines.

NHS Scotland, 2011. Code of Conduct for Healthcare Support Workers.

Nursing and Midwifery Council, 2015a. The Code: Professional Standards of Practice and Behavior for Nurses and Midwives. Nursing and Midwifery Council, London.

Nursing and Midwifery Council, 2015b. Revalidation: How to Revalidate with the NMC. Requirements for Renewing Your Registration. Nursing and Midwifery Council, London.

Nursing and Midwifery Council, 2011. Statistics about Fitness to Practice Hearings. Nursing and Midwifery Council, London.

Royal College of Nursing, 2017a. Understanding Benchmarking: RCN Guidance for Nursing Staff Working with Children and Young People. RCN, London.

Royal College of Nursing, 2017b. Safe and Effective Staffing: Nursing against the Odds. RCN, London.

Royal College of Nursing, 2008. Health Care Assistants and Assistant Practitioners: Delegation and Accountability. RCN, London.

Thompson, D., Wright, K., 2003. Developing a Unified Patient Record: A Practical Guide. Radcliffe Medical Press, Oxon.

FURTHER READING

Fernandez, R., 2016. Help Your Team Manage Stress, Anxiety and Burnout. Harvard Business Review. Jan 21.

Finnigan, M.A., Marshall, S.D., Flanagan, B.T., 2010. ISBAR for clear communication: one hospital's experience spreading the message. Australian Health Review 34 (4), 400–404.

Healthcare Commission, 2009. Investigation into Mid Staffordshire NHS Foundation Trust.

Ryley, N., Barton, D., 2015. A framework to support the revalidation process. Nursing Standard 21 (10), 16–22.

Chapter 6

Manage Your Budget

If you manage a ward or department, then you also manage a budget. You are the most appropriate person to ensure this money is used appropriately and effectively. You best understand what the needs of the patients are on your ward, and the demands on your staff. Only you can decide on the different mix of bands and skills required within your team. And only you have an idea about the amount of equipment and consumables required.

Some ward managers say that their clinical duties are more important than the budget, but it is the budget that determines what you can and cannot do clinically. How well the budget is managed directly affects how good the care is on your ward.

6.1 KNOW WHAT YOUR BUDGET IS

It typically costs in excess of £1 million per year to run a ward. The amount obviously varies depending on the number of beds and speciality. Most ward managers claim they manage a budget, but few can say what their budget is when asked. Do you know what your budget is? It is very important you are aware of how much money you are responsible for, and where and how it should be spent.

The actual figure will be shown on your monthly budget statement. It is the total amount at the bottom of the column marked 'ANNUAL BUDGET'. The budget is usually much bigger for areas such as intensive care units and accident and emergency departments.

6.1.1 Are You Managing or Just Monitoring?

Having such a large amount of money is quite a responsibility but some make the mistake of assuming that checking through the monthly statements is all that is required. This is not managing the budget, it is simply monitoring it.

Actively managing a budget entails:

- planning how next year's budget will be spent;
- keeping to specific guidelines for allocating annual leave, sickness and study leave allowances;
- performing regular staffing, skill mix and workload reviews;
- being fully involved in the yearly business planning process, which includes identifying cost pressures and service developments and writing business cases where necessary.

6.1.2 Your Staffing Establishment

Staffing costs should be regularly revised following any changes in workload. There are several off-the-shelf tools currently in use for reviewing skill mix, such as Q-Acuity (Qualitiva, 2011) and the Safer Nursing Care Tool (NHS Institute for Innovation and Improvement, 2009). These tools calculate the patients' care requirements in terms of staff numbers and grade mix. The measurements determine the ideal numbers and types of staff required per shift or the ideal numbers per group of beds, e.g. one nurse to five beds. A skill mix review will not automatically get you more staff, unfortunately. You need to get involved in the commissioning and business planning cycle to be able to influence your staffing levels (see Chapter 6).

Currently, many nurse managers use their own in-house criteria to determine their staffing numbers, such as:

● no less than two registered nurses per shift;
● no less than three staff on nights;
● one extra registered nurse each shift for 'theatre days', etc.

The nurse manager's intuition and common sense with regard to staffing requirements are often far better than any skill mix review.

6.1.3 Ratio of Nurses to Patients

In California (United States) and Victoria (Australia), the mandatory requirement for the number of nurses to patients on medical/surgical wards is 1:5 plus one in charge (International Council of Nurses (ICN), 2009). In 2016, Wales became the first country in Europe to introduce safe staffing laws for nursing. The Nurse Staffing Levels (Wales) Act places a legal duty on Health Boards and NHS Trusts in Wales to ensure they employ enough nurses to provide sensitive patient care in all settings and specifically an appropriate number of nurses are on shift in adult care settings.

Aiken et al. (2012, 2014, 2016, 2018) and Ball (2010) have studied the impact of nurse staff extensively in numerous countries and found one additional patient added to nurses' work is associated with, among other risks, a 6%–9% increase in readmissions for patients with pneumonia, heart failure and acute myocardial infarctions. Each patient added to a nurse's workload is associated with a 7% increase in risk-adjusted mortality following general surgery. The corollary was that for every 10% increase in the proportion of professional nurses among all nursing care personnel at the bedside was associated with 11% lower odds of mortality after general surgery.

In England, for example, Aiken et al. found the average patient-to-nurse ratio for all hospitals was 8.6 but varied 5.6 patients-per-nurse to 11.5 patients-per-nurse and found similarly wide variation in patient-to-nurse ratios across hospitals in every country studied. The RCN recommendation is that ward establishments should comprise 65% registered nurses and 35% healthcare assistants (HCAs) (RCN, 2006), so bear this in mind when reviewing your staffing levels with your line manager and finance advisor. This may change further with the introduction of the new nurse associate role in England, although the other three countries of the United Kingdom have declared they have no plans to introduce this role.

It is important to incident report any unsafe staffing ratios. This not only gives you an audit trail of challenges being faced with regard to staffing, but it will also be seen by other members of the hospital's senior teams. The NMC code states quite clearly that 'you must report your concerns in writing if problems in the environment of care are putting people at risk' (Nursing and Midwifery Council (NMC), 2015). In England, the NHS Constitution states that patients have a right to be treated by 'appropriately qualified and experienced staff' and, in addition, demonstrating sufficient staffing is a requirement for registration with the Care Quality Commission (CQC, 2010; Department of Health, 2010).

That noted, an added layer of complexity comes from the results of the 'Brexit' referendum in June 2016 in which the United Kingdom voted by a narrow margin (<2%) to leave the European Union of which it had been a member for the previous 40 years. It led, directly and indirectly, to a dramatic 87% reduction in the number of EU nurses joining the NMC register and an overall net loss of nurses in the United Kingdom on the nursing register for the first time ever (NMC, 2018). Substantial and enduring real-terms cuts to NHS funding, along with an ageing workforce and ageing population, have also placed a strain on existing staff, and an important part of your role includes providing the larger context of the workforce in which your team works.

6.1.4 Matching the Roster to Your Staffing Establishment

Your staffing establishment is worked out by your finance advisor using information from your roster (i.e. the minimum staffing levels required per shift that either you have identified personally or through a formal skill mix review). It is essential that the minimum staffing levels on your roster match the numbers in your staffing establishment. If you do not know for sure, ask your finance advisor to work it out for you.

Each directorate usually has a dedicated finance advisor. It is their job to work with you to help you ensure the budget is right for your needs. It is your job to maintain regular contact with them. If you do not, who is it they are getting their information from? And how accurate is that information?

6.2 PRIORITISE PAY

Your budget is made up of two parts:

1. PAY – this section reflects the salaries of your staff.
2. NON-PAY – this section contains the money for equipment and consumables.

The PAY section takes up the first part of your budget statement. It is the part that you need to concentrate on because it usually comprises at least 80% of your total budget.

6.2.1 The Importance of Good Roster Management

If your PAY budget is overspent, it can be due to inefficient rosters. To manage the PAY part of your budget effectively, you need to:

- ensure your staffing establishment matches your required 'numbers' on the roster;
- manage the 20%–23% allowance, which covers annual leave, study leave and unplanned absence such as sick leave;
- control agency and bank usage to within the 20%–23% allowance.

The use of bank and agency nursing is closely monitored throughout organisations; however, there does need to be a balance between budget use and patient safety. Do not be afraid to push for the use of bank or agency, if it could impact on patient safety.

6.2.1.1 Staffing Establishment

You will probably have set minimum staffing levels for each shift over a 7-day week (Table 6.1). The person who does the roster then allocates the staff to meet those minimum levels on each shift. Your staffing establishment (which you should receive with your monthly statement) is worked out based on your set shift requirements (Table 6.2). You must check regularly with your finance advisor that they match up. If you do not ensure that the staffing establishment meets the set shift numbers, then you cannot devise the roster within budget and are therefore failing to manage it.

6.2.1.2 20%–23% Absence Allowance (Which Should Be Built Into Your Establishment)

When your finance advisor works out your staffing requirements, they use your roster numbers but also put in an additional 20%–23% to cover annual leave, sickness/absence and study leave. It means that your final staffing establishment

TABLE 6.1 Example of Minimum Staffing Levels Over a 7-Day Week

	Monday	Tuesday	Wednesday	Thursday	Friday	Saturday	Sunday
Early	6	7	6	6	6	5	5
Late	6	6	6	6	5	5	5
Night	4	4	4	4	4	3	3

TABLE 6.2 Example of a Ward-Staffing Establishment

Description	Budget (WTE)	Actual (WTE)
Ward manager (band 7)	1.0	1.0
Sister/charge nurse (band 6)	2.0	1.8
Staff nurse (band 5)	12.0	12.2
HCA (band 4)	8.0	6.0
HCA (band 3)	5.0	7.0
Ward clerk	1.0	1.0
TOTAL	29	29

HCA, healthcare assistant; *WTE*, whole time equivalent.
1.00 WTE is full time, < 1.00 WTE is part time.

should provide you with enough to cover your annual leave, sickness/absence and study leave requirements and remain within budget.

Sometimes some of this allowance is separated as a separate line within your budget statement and labelled as 'bank/agency costs'.

The additional 20%–23% usually comprises:

- 13.5% annual leave and bank holidays ($27 + 8 = 35$ days)
- 1%–2% study leave (2.5–5 days)
- 5%–7% unplanned absences such as sickness, maternity, compassionate and carers leave (13–18 days)

If you do not manage annual leave, sick leave and study leave correctly, you can overspend unnecessarily. Check out with your finance advisor exactly what percentage your organisation adds to cover absence allowance. Without knowing this figure, you cannot manage your PAY budget effectively.

6.2.1.3 Bank and Agency Usage

Use bank (NHS Professionals in England) instead of agency wherever possible. They cost little more than permanent staff and are often comprised of already permanent staff members looking for extra shifts. If you are sent an agency nurse because no bank nurses are available, an additional 33% is usually charged in commission to the agency. This means that for every three shifts covered by agency staff, one shift should remain unfilled in order to make up for the extra cost. Obviously, this needs to be handled very carefully because, at the same time, you cannot compromise patient care. Some compensate for the extra commission charges by booking agency nurses for a 'half shift' only.

In some organisations, the most popular shifts for bank staff are early shifts. This means that the late and night shifts are covered by the agency. It therefore makes sense to compile rosters to ensure that most late and your own staff, leaving the vacant shifts mainly as early shifts, cover night shifts. This will ensure that there is a higher chance of getting bank staff rather than agency.

6.2.2 'Buddy up' With Another Ward

Try and work closely with another ward manager and share staff between your two wards during the hard times. It is advisable to link up with another ward or department with a similar speciality within your directorate for the purpose of sharing staff. You could meet with the manager once per week to go through the following week or month's roster. This enables you to identify areas where resources could be shared and to plan ahead for expected shortfalls. It is important to communicate with your staff that they may be changing between wards. Ensure that staff that are being asked to move feel confident in looking after the patients they are allocated.

6.2.3 Be Flexible With Your Staffing Establishment

Be more flexible with your staffing establishment. If you are unable to recruit a certain grade of staff into your vacant post, then consider other options. Can you replace with a different grade of staff? Think carefully; perhaps it would be better to employ an available lower grade of staff rather than fill the vacancy continually with bank and agency.

As the budget holder, you do not have to stick to the grades of staff in your budget statement. You can adjust them according to the needs of the ward and what is available so long as you remain within budget. Your finance advisor's role is to assist you in doing so and they will calculate any differences for you. You will also need your line manager's overall approval.

6.3 GO THROUGH YOUR MONTHLY BUDGET STATEMENT

The budget statement tells what you have spent. It is like going through your own bank statement at the end of the month; nothing should come as a surprise. It should confirm what you already know.

The layout of the budget statement varies between organisations. However, the information contained is basically the same. It is usually divided into two parts, PAY and NON-PAY, and is best read using the following columns.

6.3.1 Establishment (Budget)

This column tells you how many staff you can employ within your budget (WTE stands for 'whole time equivalent': 1.0 WTE is full time, and anything less than 1.0 WTE is part time (e.g. 0.6 WTE equates to funding for someone to work 3 days per week)).

6.3.2 Establishment (Actual)

This column tells you how many staff you have in post. The numbers will vary. For example, if you cannot recruit up to establishment in band 6, you can recruit more in band 5 to compensate, as long as the final salary figure remains the same.

6.3.3 Code

This is the finance code given to each particular grade of staff or type of equipment. The first part of the code relates to your ward (usually a 4-digit number). The second part relates to the category of staff or equipment (usually another 4-digit number).

6.3.4 Annual Budget

This is usually the last column on the right-hand side of your budget statement. The numbers in this column never change. It tells you what money you have to spend over the whole year. You should be very familiar with these figures.

6.3.5 Current Month's Budget, Expenditure and Variance

These three columns tell you what you had to spend in the last month (budget), what you did spend (expenditure) and what the difference is (variance).

6.3.6 Year to Date's Budget, Expenditure and Variance

These three columns tell you what you have had in your budget so far since the beginning of the financial year (budget), what you have spent in that time (expenditure) and where you are at the moment in terms of overall underspend or overspend (variance).

6.3.7 Checking Through the Columns

When you receive your budget statement, the first thing you need to do is check the total amount in the 'year to date' variance column. It tells you how overspent or underspent you are at the moment. Remember to concentrate on the PAY section, as this is usually the part where most of your budget is allocated. When moving into a more senior management role, you may find that understanding budgets is overwhelming. It is important to remember to use the resources around you – use your Director of nursing, your financial advisor, etc. to help make sense of the information in front of you; asking questions is not a weakness, it shows that you are willing to ask for help.

If you have an overspend first of all, do not panic, take a look at the rest of this column to find out which bit is overspent. Overspends should not be a surprise. You know when you have used extra agency to cover high sickness levels or have had an unexpected increase in workload in the past month. The key to managing your budget effectively is deciding what to do about this overspend. You should have already warned your line manager and finance manager, and together worked out a plan of action to bring the budget back in line. If not, it is advisable to do so at this point.

You also need to check the first two columns in the PAY section (i.e. budgeted and actual establishment) for accuracy. It is often the case that a 'leavers' form may not have been processed when a member of staff leaves or transfers to another ward. If this happens, your ward will continue to fund their pay until the form is processed.

Overall, your main task with the budget statement is to check for any inaccuracies and identify the main variances. You should then discuss your findings with your financial advisor each month and write a plan of action for the coming month.

6.3.8 Involve Your Team

Go through your budget statement with your staff regularly. Get feedback from those who have responsibility for aspects of the NON-PAY. Often, housekeepers have a better idea of stock levels and ordering processes than the coordinators do. Utilise their experience and ask them for advice on where we could reduce expenditure on stock that may not be used often or ask them to look at cheaper alternatives.

Ask staff if they have any innovative ideas to help reduce expenditure, something as simple as changing the type of dressing used for equally effective but less expensive ones can save thousands of pounds a year. Bearing in mind the biggest demand on your budget is staff costs, ask them where savings could be made in their time by increasing efficiency and in practice not wasting their most precious resource, their time, on activities that do not add value to them or patients. Examples can include looking for observation machines that are placed randomly around the ward, instead of having a 'home' where they are always placed, completing excessive paperwork, etc. While their pay will not change and will not release cash, it is a cost avoidance as it reduces the cost of the wasted effort by releasing time to care instead of chasing their tails around the unit.

Discuss and agree on actions for both PAY and NON-PAY; sharing the budget statements with your team helps in their development and ensures they appreciate the links between good budgeting and good patient care.

6.4 MANAGE ANNUAL LEAVE

6.4.1 Calculating the Annual Leave Allowance per Roster

The average percentage given for annual leave is usually 13.5%. This equates to 35 days (27 + 8) per person. In order to manage this annual leave allowance effectively, you have to make sure that a certain number of staff are on annual leave at any one time. Generally, 13.5% of your establishment equates to around one in every seven staff. In other words, for every seven staff in your team, one should be on annual leave. This ensures that annual leave is spread throughout the year so that adequate numbers of staff are available to work at all times.

6.4.2 Spreading Annual Leave Throughout the Year

Poor staffing levels between January and March due to high levels of annual leave indicate that the ward manager has not managed their budget properly, leading to an overspend as a consequence. Encourage your staff to take annual leave regularly throughout the year and book this at least 4 weeks in advance of the roster. The following guidelines are generally recommended (check with your local organisational guidelines):

- By end-June – minimum of 1 week must have been taken.
- By end-September – minimum of 3 weeks must have been taken.
- By end-December – minimum of 5 weeks must have been taken.
- Jan to end-March – maximum of 1 week of annual leave to be taken.

A good tip is to keep an annual leave planner on the wall in the ward office with separate annual leave lines for the number of staff who can take annual leave at any one time. Staff can then fill in the slots where they want to take annual leave over the coming year. You can also see at a glance what is happening and be able to intervene if necessary. It will stop staff leaving it to the last minute to book and finding out there are no annual leave slots left.

If any of your staff wish to carry annual leave allowance over into the next financial year, you should clarify first how you can allow for this within the following year's budget.

Try not to resort to allocating annual leave. It is better to take time to explain to your team how the budget and annual leave allowance are so closely linked. Get them to understand that if they do not book their annual leave early and spread it out over the year, it will cause an overspend in the budget and you will end up having to make other cutbacks (e.g. stopping bank and agency) to bring it back in line. Another reason why it is important that staff take regular periods of leave is patient safety as tired staff are more likely to make mistakes.

6.5 MANAGE YOUR UNPLANNED ABSENCE ALLOWANCE

You usually have an allowance of up to 7% for unplanned absence such as sick leave, maternity leave, carers leave, etc. (check what your own organisation allows): 7% equates to around 18 days of unplanned absence per person per year without incurring an overspend. This does not mean that each person can take 18 days off sick per year! It means that you have enough funding to cover an overall absence rate (due to sickness, maternity, carers or compassionate leave) in your team of up to 7% without going over budget.

Make sure you have systems in place to monitor sickness rates closely. You need to be able to look at trends over time. It is not enough to get a 'feel' for the level of absence. Calculate it at the end of each completed roster. In some organisations, particularly those using e-rostering, the ward managers are sent a summary of their staff sickness rates each month. If your organisation does not have this system in place, you can easily work it out for yourself using the equation outlined in Box 6.1.

On completion of each 4-week roster, it is advisable to keep and update a continuous record of the team's sickness rates (Table 6.3).

6.5.1 Sickness Monitoring

You should be able to demonstrate that you are taking action where sickness levels are high. If the sickness rates go beyond your organisation's target level, you need to look at the reasons and take action to reduce them. If the main reason for sickness is due to back problems, for example, then it would be wise to undertake further moving and handling risk assessments, involve the manual handling advisor and invest extra funding into moving and handling training/equipment.

BOX 6.1 Calculating Staff Sickness Rates

Number of days lost ÷ number of days rostered × 100 = sickness percentage.
Example: If Nurse Smith was rostered to work 20 days during the last roster but was off sick for four of them:

$4 \div 20 \times 100 = 20\%$

The time lost by Nurse Smith was 20% of her potential working time.

TABLE 6.3 Example of Record of Staff Sickness on Ward at 6 Months

Staff	Shifts Rostered	Shifts Off Sick	% Sickness	Episodes
Rose	120	6	5	3
Emma	122	8	6.5	2
Jane	120	2	1.7	1
Susan	119	0	0	0
Amy	120	5	4.2	1
Gemma	121	0	0	0
Dave	120	2	1.7	1
John	100	0	0	0
Total	942	23	2.4	8

Total number of shifts lost to sickness ÷ total number of shifts rostered = 23 ÷ 942 × 100.
Total percentage of sickness to date = 2.4%.

6.5.2 Maternity/Parental Leave

The percentage for unplanned absence usually incorporates parental leave. If the parental leave is particularly high within your department, you need to highlight this with your general manager who will have the authority to transfer funding between departments if necessary.

Some organisations hold the maternity leave budget centrally. If this is the case, you must ensure the allowance is allocated to your budget when affected by parental leave. This can be achieved through close liaison and monitoring with your line manager and finance advisor.

6.5.3 Other Leaves

With the increasing emphasis on family-friendly and flexible working policies, there are now other types of leave that you need to manage carefully within your allowance for unplanned absences. These include time off to attend antenatal classes, adoption leave, carer's leave and compassionate leave. Keep a running check on how much all this leave is costing you. You may have to apply for more to be added in your budget.

6.6 PLAN YOUR STUDY LEAVE ALLOWANCE

You usually have an allowance within the budget of around 1%–2% for covering study leave (some organisations allocate more, some less, so you must check exactly what you have with your finance advisor). This equates to between 2 and 5 days per staff member per year. This does not mean that each member of your team is entitled to be released for this number of study days per year. The study leave allowance should be viewed as a total for the whole team of staff. For example, if you have a team of 30 WTE, 2% study leave allowance would give you up to 150 study days per year that can be granted to your team ($30 \times 5 = 150$ days).

The study leave allowance needs to be planned carefully at around November time in the preceding financial year, taking the following steps:

1. Multiply the total number of your budgeted WTE establishment by the number of study days your organisation allocates per WTE, which will give the total number of days that can be allocated for study leave over the coming financial year (as outlined in the example above).
2. Identify all the study needs of all staff in your team (via the annual appraisal process) in terms of mandatory requirements plus professional and personal development needs.
3. Find out exactly what the study leave requirements are for each course that staff members have identified.
4. Total the amount of study leave that your staff will require for the coming year.

5. If the total study leave required is more than the total number of shifts allowed in your budget, priorities have to be made. A good way to decide these priorities is to ask your team. Use a team meeting to get them to decide among themselves who gets priority. Facilitate the discussion to ensure it is done in a fair and consistent manner.

It is always advisable to keep a portion of the study leave allowance aside to be used for unexpected courses, workshops, conferences or seminars that may arise throughout the year, which would benefit the staff and service. If extra courses come up during the year that do not come within the 1%–2% allowance, replacement costs must be identified from another source, unless the workload means you can 'go down' on numbers, or the member of staff concerned is willing to go in their own (unpaid) time. Education funding currently is severely reduced; it is important that staff are supported and guided as to how they can find funding for any courses that would be beneficial for them.

6.6.1 Other Sources of Funding

Keep close links with the manager of your organisation's training and development department and with your link university. This will help keep you aware of any further 'pots' of money that become available throughout the year (often at the end of each financial year between January and March). Various charities such as the League of Friends will sometimes support staff for training courses. You have to find out where these extra funds are; they tend not to be generally advertised.

6.6.2 Mandatory Training

Include all mandatory training within your allowance. If you are not careful, mandatory training days can use up all your study leave allowance. The staff in the training department may not realise this. It is up to you and your colleagues to point it out to them and present an alternative solution. Some organisations have condensed their training into short 2-h sessions, which can either be put together to cover three to four subjects in 1 day or held as separate sessions during the afternoon handover period.

Study leave needs to be carefully controlled. Keeping your staff informed and fully involved in the process of allocation helps them to understand the restrictions you are working to and reduces any feelings of resentment about study leave allocation.

6.7 GET YOUR STAFF INVOLVED IN NON-PAY

The NON-PAY part of your budget is usually set out in the second part of your budget statement. The only difference between PAY and NON-PAY on the statement is that the establishment and WTE columns will remain blank because NON-PAY does not involve people. The overall amount you have in NON-PAY is usually far less than the PAY section. The list of items may be longer, but this does not mean it is more important. It is just easier to ascertain where the money has gone.

NON-PAY may appear to be your lower priority but it still needs tight control. A good way to manage it is to delegate each budget line to a member of your staff. This will give them a good insight into budget management and help them to develop budgeting skills with appropriate support. The main ones to delegate are pharmacy/drugs, medical supplies and stationery. These usually have another separate list showing more minute details of the expenditure that your staff can manage, leaving you to concentrate on the PAY budget, which is your biggest expenditure.

6.7.1 Pharmacy/Drugs

The nurse responsible for this budget would probably form close links with the ward pharmacist. Their role would include going through the monthly pharmacy budget in detail and becoming familiar with what is being used, what is needed and any changes that are being made. They would be able to identify any cost pressures (see Chapter 6), such as new routine drugs introduced during the current financial year that were not originally budgeted for.

6.7.2 Medical Supplies

Most hospitals nowadays rely on a top-up system. Allocating one member of your team to monitor usage and trends will help keep the stock levels appropriate to what is needed and identify any unnecessary expenditure. They will also be able to liaise with the appropriate company representatives (alongside NHS supplies if working within the NHS) to keep abreast of what is new and perhaps more appropriate for your group of patients.

6.7.3 Stationery

The stationery budget is often best delegated to your ward receptionist who is usually the most appropriate person to know what is being used and where to make savings.

6.8 BE MORE ACTIVE IN THE BUSINESS PLANNING PROCESS

Get involved with the business planning process for your directorate. The budgets are reset each year as part of the annual business planning process cycle (which in turn takes account of predicted levels of activity and decisions made by the commissioning groups). It is something with which you should be familiar as the budget holder. Some ward managers are left out of this important process. It is up to you to make sure you get involved. Ward budgets can be inappropriate if someone else is deciding what your ward needs.

The process usually begins around November every year in the NHS when all wards and departments in your organisation have to identify what they need for the next year. The whole process takes up to 6 months (remember, each financial year is from 1 April to 31 March). The general manager's role is to produce the final business plan that represents all the wards and departments in their directorate. The final plan outlines to the board what funding is required to manage the service in the coming year. It includes any extra funding required due to changes in the service.

The director of finance together with the other board directors agree how much each directorate will get based on the business plans which the general managers have submitted, and the levels of activity and decisions made by the trust's commissioners. It is the general manager's role to write the full business plan, not yours. You are a nurse manager, not a business manager. However, you do need to contribute to the process.

6.8.1 The Business Plan

Your general manager is usually tasked with identifying the *cost pressures* and *service developments* through all their department leads:

- A *cost pressure* is an approved change that has already happened over the past year, which needs funding for the future to *maintain existing service levels*, e.g. equipment that requires updating/replacing or a nationally approved pay rise for staff.
- A *service development* is an authorised planned change that will be needed to *improve the quantity or quality of service* in the future, e.g. the implementation of a patient follow-up service or the appointment of a nurse specialist.

The general manager usually has to produce evidence for each item in the form of a business case. This is the stage where you need to ensure you are not left out. If you need another member of staff due to increased turnover of patients, then you have to present a 'business case'. Do this together with your line manager and finance advisor, who will work out all the costs for you.

If you do not do this, either:

- someone else will do it for you; this might be someone who may not understand the service as well as you and therefore will not present your case so well or
- your needs will not be added to the overall business plan.

There are usually too many cost pressures and service developments, so priorities have to be made. Some will be rejected because there is simply not enough money for them all. If you are not involved and do not get across to your general manager the importance of your needs, then you will probably not get them.

6.8.2 How to Write a Business Case

There is no point in writing a business case if:

- your manager does not agree and has no intention of agreeing to include it in the overall business plan or
- your manager feels that the funding could be sought elsewhere.

A business case is simply a way of presenting evidence that the item is really needed. Many organisations provide a business case form to be completed in each case. Box 6.2 gives an example of the information that is generally required.

6.9 DO NOT DO ANYTHING WITHOUT IDENTIFIED FUNDING

It is imperative that you do not implement anything new without the identified funding. As mentioned previously, nurses have a wonderful ability to cope when under-resourced. Unfortunately, this can lead to more problems than it solves. If you can take on extra work without extra resources, then why would the organisation give you further funding?

If you are already providing an extra service without extra funding, you have to take action to ensure the funding is put into the following year's budget. For example, if you have a couple of HCAs who have automatically been given a pay increase for achieving NVQ level 3, but no budget had been set aside for this, it would be classified as a cost pressure. In the meantime, look at what service you will cease to provide in order to provide the extra service within budget. For example, you can alter the staffing establishment to meet the extra cost of the HCAs' increased salary.

Always involve your finance advisor. Being refused a cost pressure does not give you the automatic right to overspend because you have the service anyway. You have to make savings elsewhere within your budget.

6.9.1 Get It in Writing

Do not take on extra work with verbal promises of extra funding; ensure you have some sort of written confirmation. It is not uncommon for ward managers to open extra beds or be persuaded to provide staff cover for clinics on the promise that funding will follow, only to find that the funding never materialises. The new service soon becomes established and cannot be withdrawn or patient care

BOX 6.2 Example of a Format for Writing a Business Case

Title

Explain as fully as you can within the title. Include the cost here (e.g. replacement ECG machine @ £5000 or 1 × band 5 nurse @ £30,000).

Introduction

Give a brief summary of what the problem is, the solution, why and what is the cost. Ensure you state clearly how much this initial outlay will save you in the long term.

Background

Explain the background but remember that non-clinical people may be reviewing this, so you should assume that they know little about it. Explain what the benefits will be and what will happen if you do not get it. Your case will be much stronger if you can relate it to government targets, policy or standards (e.g. CQC, Commissioning for Quality and Innovation (CQUIN)). Also include risk assessment results where possible. In England, all business plans should link with the Operating Framework, which is a set of national priorities issued by the Department of Health and Social Care each year.

Options Analysis

First, describe your current service and then list all the options that could be taken, and for each of them give a brief outline including advantages, risk, constraints, potential impact, outcomes and decision (i.e. accept/reject with reasons). If possible, include a cost-benefit analysis (e.g. what would the more expensive one provide as opposed to the cheaper version?). Include the option of no change. What would happen if you do nothing? Try to talk in numbers as much as possible (e.g. how much it would cost in terms of nursing hours spent going round other wards each day to borrow an ECG machine). Your finance advisor will work out the costings for you. How many patients would suffer? How many may have treatment delayed? What care standard will you not meet?

Preferred Option

State your preferred option and say why. Also list all the items that make up your final cost figure. Do not forget to include time and people. Include any savings that will be made (e.g. reduced cost of calling out facilities to fix the ECG machine every few weeks, reduced re-admission rates with an extra member of staff). It is your finance advisor's role to work out the costs for you.

Recommendations

Conclude with your recommendation(s).

will suffer, so do not let yourself get into such a situation. Becoming wise to the business planning process reduces the risk of being duped into taking on work without appropriate funding.

If it does happen (e.g. your line manager may have agreed on your behalf to a change without realising the extra work involved and it is too late for the decision to be reversed), you should take action quickly by identifying which aspects of your existing workload must be cut in order to provide the new service. Let your manager know your decision in writing and do not try to cope and allow your staff to become exhausted and stressed by trying to provide extra services without the appropriate resources.

6.10 MEET REGULARLY WITH YOUR FINANCE ADVISOR

It is essential that you meet with your financial advisor regularly to do the following:

1. *Ensure that any inaccuracies in your budget are rectified.* If you have been charged for something that you have not used, it is your financial advisor's role to get the money transferred back to your budget, but you have to identify it first. Unprocessed 'starters' and 'leavers' forms are a common source of inaccuracies that need to be identified and corrected quickly.
2. *Ensure that your staffing establishment always matches the limits set on your roster.* This is essential for good budget management. Each time a member of your staff resigns, review the job with your team, do not always replace 'like with like' as the workload or skill requirement may have changed. Your finance advisor will be able to advise how you could achieve the change within your current staffing establishment but still remain within budget.
3. *Check that you are using bank and agency wisely.* If you are using them just to cover staff vacancies, there should be no overspend. If you are using bank and agency to cover sickness, there should not be an overspend unless your sickness levels are above the sickness allowance that was added to your budget.
4. *Calculate and prepare for any predicted overspends.* Obviously, there will be unforeseen costs such as an outbreak of MRSA or a patient who requires one-to-one care for some time. These types of extra costs are not included within your budget, but you do need to monitor them closely. Simply saying 'we are overspent because it has been busy' is insufficient. It will appear that you are not managing your budget properly. It is far better to report that 'we have a predicted overspend of £6000 this month due to the extra staffing required to special a high-dependency patient for 7 days because there were no available beds in HDU'. You must see your finance advisor early so they can forecast the extra cost to your budget. You can then work together with them and your line manager to plan how you can get your budget back on line over the rest of the financial year.
5. *Help you prepare a business case should you require more staff or equipment.* Remember that you will need your general manager's agreement before you go ahead and compile a business case.

It is the finance manager's role to provide specialist expertise and support you in managing the budget. But they will not come to you. Be proactive. Go to them and seek their advice. They are not clinically trained and often do not understand the complexities of running a ward. You are not a finance expert and do not understand the intricacies of how hospital finance works. Work together and use each other's skills to ensure your budget is managed efficiently and effectively, thus ensuring a high standard of patient care.

6.11 ACTION POINTS

- Meet with your finance advisor to confirm that your roster numbers match the staffing establishment; ensure you know the percentage of absence allowance and go through your budget statement explaining anything that you do not understand.
- Follow up with regular appointments throughout the year, preferably monthly. Go through your budget statement and discuss any problems and any changes you wish to make.
- Calculate how many staff should be on annual leave each week and ensure all future rosters are compiled with the right numbers of staff on annual leave.
- Starting from this year, plan your next year's study leave quota in advance with your team.
- If your HR team does not supply you with monthly sickness figures for your team, maintain your own records for now.
- Delegate some NON-PAY budget lines to your staff for professional development purposes, and to allow you to concentrate on PAY.
- Have a look at last year's business plan and ask your general manager to go through it with you, explaining anything you do not understand. Get involved with next year's plan and put forward your team's needs.
- Review the budget in all your team meetings. Explain and involve the team in issues such as annual leave and study leave allowances.
- Involve your staff in *all* decisions such as who gets study leave and where to make cost savings.
- Do not take on extra work without written confirmation of funding.

REFERENCES

Aiken, L.H., Cerōn, C., Simonetti, M., et al., 2018. Hospital nurse staffing and patient outcomes. Revista Médica Clínica Las Condes 29 (3), 322–327.

Aiken, L.H., Sloane, D., Griffiths, P., et al., 2016. Nursing skill mix in European hospitals: cross-sectional study of the association with mortality, patient ratings, and quality of care. BMJ Quality and Safety 26 (7), 559–568. https://doi.org/10.1136/bmjqs-2016-005567.

Aiken, L.H., Sloane, D.M., Bruyneel, L., et al., 2014. Nurse staffing and education and hospital mortality in nine European countries: a retrospective observational study. Lancet 383 (9931), 1824–1830.

Aiken, L.H., Sermeus, W., Vanden Heede, K., et al., 2012. Patient safety, satisfaction, and quality of hospital care: cross-sectional surveys of nurses and patients in 12 countries in Europe and the United States. British Medical Journal 344, e1717.

Care Quality Commission, 2010. Essential Standards of Quality and Safety. Guidance about Compliance.

Department of Health, 2010. The NHS Constitution. GRASP, 2011. Skill Mix Analysis.

International Council of Nurses, 2009. Nursing Matters Factsheet: Nurse: Patient Ratios. ICN, Geneva.

NHS Institute for Innovation and Improvement, 2009. The Safer Nursing Care Tool.

Nursing and Midwifery Council, 2018. The NMC Register. NMC, London.

Nursing and Midwifery Council, 2015. The Code: Professional Standards for Practice and Behaviour for Nurses and Midwives. NMC, London.

Qualitiva, 2011. Q-acuity Nursing Acuity Data Tool.

Royal College of Nursing, 2006. Policy Guidance 15/2006: Setting Appropriate Ward Nurse Staffing in NHS Acute Trusts. RCN.

FURTHER READING

Ball, J., 2010. Guidance on Safe Nurse Staffing Levels in the UK. RCN, London.

Chapter 7

Improve Quality and Safety

Healthcare is inherently risky, therefore managing risk involves establishing factual information. Clinical governance can often be seen as a negative term within healthcare, but it is one of the most important parts of a healthcare system. Clinical governance is established to improve clinical quality, learn from mistakes made and to monitor trends and patterns. There are many ways different areas of clinical governance are measured to help improve the quality of the work from every person within an organisation.

Clinical governance is a multifactorial entity that is not just an auditing tool for clinical errors; its role extends beyond clinical errors and covers every aspect that could potentially affect, positively or negatively, a patient's journey through the healthcare system.

Reporting and monitoring of errors is essential to improving and enhancing a patient's journey, but we must also look at the positive quality measures and expand on those.

Patient/family surveys, staff surveys, comments, complaints and incidents give us a vast amount of information about where to target resources to improve our service.

Patient-specific feedback gives you an insight into how to best improve the service from a user perspective, one that we often do not have first-hand experience of.

Staff surveys are essential to get honest feedback as to how to improve working environments for staff, as well as highlighting the positives that can be further expanded on.

This chapter explains the process of quality monitoring and improvement as well as the practical tasks of dealing with complaints and incidents.

7.1 QUALITY INDICATORS

The ultimate goal for anyone working within healthcare is to ensure the patients in their care receive the best treatment possible. To do this, we examine certain quality indicators and try to get an understanding of what is needed to improve the service. When doing this, often we find that there is a knock-on effect somewhere else. For example, the 4-h waiting target in emergency departments indirectly led to increased pressure on beds, and the initial mixing of male and female patients subsequently led to problems with privacy and dignity. This in turn led to further quality indicators being introduced for single sex wards/bays and various other initiatives for increasing privacy and dignity. Other examples include the changing of ward layouts to single rooms and four to six bed bays to meet hygiene, privacy and dignity indicators, resulting in the reduced ability of nurses to adequately observe, thereby contributing to an increased number of falls. Quality indicators introduced helped to reduce the number of falls, including initiatives such as hourly rounding.

It is important, however, to remember that, first and foremost, you are a clinician and the patients' needs are your priority. This is particularly pertinent at times when you have to choose between meeting a quality indicator and ensuring that patients get appropriate individualised care. An example would be the choice between getting a patient discharged by 12 midday or taking the time to ensure they understand their discharge medication. To be able to make an appropriate choice, you should have some idea of what the most important quality indicators are, where they come from and why they are so important. There will always be a tension between what is best for patients and what is best for the system and helping staff navigate those tensions is an important role as it helps them understand their work in the context of the wider system demands.

7.1.1 Care Quality Commission

In England, all healthcare providers – both NHS and private – must be registered with the Care Quality Commission (CQC), which has a number of quality indicators that have to be met, called the Essential Standards of Quality and Safety (CQC, 2010). If any part of your organisation does not meet these standards, the CQC has the power to suspend work or even shut down that department or care home and has done so. Before any place of work is shut down, recommendations are given to support the failing area to come up to the standard and the organisation is put into so-called 'special measures'. This provides a framework within which the CQC uses enforcement powers in response to inadequate care and work with, or signpost to, other organisations in the system to ensure improvements are made.

The systems in Scotland, Wales and Northern Ireland all vary slightly from this. For example, the Scottish Healthcare Inspectorate focuses on quality indicators for reducing infection rates and inspects each local health board twice every 3 years. NHS Wales improves quality through the 1000 Lives Plus programme and through locally agreed targets.

Many of the quality indicators used are heavily influenced by the National Institute for Health and Clinical Excellence (NICE) guidance in England and Wales. Scotland and Northern Ireland differ in that they usually (but not always) disseminate the NICE guidance but only after reviewing it first.

CQC visits can often cause great amounts of unintended anxiety for all members of the team. It is important to support your staff during any inspections and to give them knowledge as to how inspections are run and what may be asked of them.

Ultimately, unless it is shown to be failing or requiring improvement, how your department is run should not change. The standards expected from the CQC are what should be embedded in the care the team already provides. Even if the standards are embedded, there are always certain aspects that some people will be concerned over, whether this is being interviewed or simply from not understanding the formalities of an inspection.

Some hospitals now run a mock CQC visit, interviewing staff and using CQC frameworks to conduct informal inspections. This peer system means that people from the same trust, but external to the department or directorate, can give honest feedback in areas that may need improvement before an official visit.

If you are unsure as to whether initiatives as this are run within your organisation, speak with your manager to find out. If not, suggest it as a quality improvement project.

The CQC values are easily accessed on their website and will give you a framework to help with any improvement works that you may need to carry out.

7.1.2 Commissioning for Quality and Innovation

In addition to the CQC performance indicators in England, commissioning groups also set certain quality indicators to be met. Commissioning for Quality and Innovations (CQUINs) were initially developed and introduced into the NHS in England in 2009. The premise behind the introduction was to help further improve quality and drive innovation. This was done by making some income conditional on an improvement in care within certain areas.

Commissioned services in hospitals are attached to quality indicators specifically for the service commissioned. If the quality indicators are not met, the commissioning bodies can potentially withhold a percentage of the total payment.

Some of the quality indicators used, for example, can include areas such as the percentage of patients who have had a venous thromboembolism risk assessment on admission, the percentage of 12-noon discharges and the percentage of surgical site infections.

This results in both national and local targets being set to help improve the quality and safety of patient care.

7.2 IDENTIFY MISTAKES AND RISKS

There will always be an element of risk within any healthcare system, yet risk is predominantly seen in a negative light. This is not to say that risk does not have negatives, but without risk, we would never have innovations or improvements.

Managing risk has two major purposes. First, to reduce harm coming to people involved within a task, be this staff, patients, visitors or external agencies. Second, it is to empower and support people to push for innovation and improvement in the care they are providing.

Managing risk is therefore a continuous process. Standards, policies and procedures are continually being updated to reduce the risk of things going wrong but inevitably no system or human being is perfect, and mistakes will continue to be made. What is important is how we learn and adapt from mistakes.

We currently have a National Reporting and Learning System (NRLS) originally set up by the National Patient Safety Agency (NPSA) in 2003, which gathers data from all healthcare organisations in relation to patient safety incidents in England and Wales (Northern Ireland and Scotland operate more local systems of reporting and data collection). All information submitted is analysed to identify hazards, risks and opportunities to continuously improve the safety of patient care. The NRLS distributes this learning from data via patient safety alerts, guidelines and policies.

Each NHS organisation also has a form of dealing with complaints that ensures they are investigated locally, recurring themes are identified, and improvements are made accordingly. These are often known as adverse incident report forms and can have different names dependent on the individual system used within each trust.

As the ward manager, you should be familiar with the systems for dealing with complaints and incidents. This will ensure that you are able to support your staff and the patients and relatives involved and focus on making improvements to care as a direct result.

Incident reporting should be encouraged and not be seen as a negative process. Ultimately, each report submitted gives insight in to areas where improvements could be made. Involve all team members in incidents to give them a greater understanding of the reporting, management and learning. This can help to alleviate stress and anxiety if they are ever involved in one.

7.2.1 Be Open and Do Not Be Afraid to Say Sorry

We have previously spoken about the impact of saying sorry in Chapter 3; however, it is important to reiterate this message when talking about risk and quality improvement.

When mistakes are made, early explanation of the situation and a genuine apology can ultimately be enough for patients and families to feel their concern is being taken seriously and that lessons will be learnt. 'When things do go wrong, an apology can be a powerful remedy; simple to deliver and costing nothing' (Parliamentary and Health Service Ombudsman, 2010).

Saying sorry is not an admission of liability (NHS Litigation Authority (NHSLA), 2009); in fact, there have been various studies from hospitals in Australia, Singapore and the United States that have shown a marked reduction in the number of claims since policies were introduced that promote the concept of saying sorry when things go wrong (NPSA, 2009). Most organisations now have guidelines for staff on how to communicate with patients and their families when a mistake has been made, particularly when any harm has been caused. One recommendation for ensuring a good apology is to refer to the three R's recommended by Armstrong (2010):

- Regret – say sorry.
- Reason – be honest and explain that it was unintentional.
- Remedy – explain the next steps such as investigation and feedback.

7.2.1.1 Duty of Candour

Many of us working within the UK healthcare service will be aware of the tragic events that unfolded at the Mid Staffordshire NHS Trust in which serious system and leadership failings, over a number of years, led to at least 400 more deaths than might have been expected. Following these events, an inquiry was undertaken, and Sir Robert Francis QC produced several volumes of what became known as The Francis Report (2013). This is essential reading for anyone working within healthcare.

One of the most positive and fundamental recommendations produced from this report was the introduction of duty of candour reports. This recommendation was adopted by the CQC and is an essential part of all healthcare systems.

In short, duty of candour is simply to ensure that all healthcare professionals must be open, honest and transparent when things go wrong, not only to patients and their families but also to the organisation itself.

Many people new to managerial roles may find duty of candour a daunting experience; however, you will never go through a duty of candour on your own. Duty of candour is a process that should be undertaken by the entire multidisciplinary team. As a multidisciplinary team, you will have the support of multiple experience levels and this will help to relive some of the pressure you may feel. Often, most trusts offer training on the management of duty of candour to help give you an understanding of the process; if you are new to the process, it is worth investing the time to attend. The Nursing and Midwifery Council (2018) states the following:

(a) Your duty is to be open and honest with patients in your care, or those close to them, if something goes wrong.
(b) Your duty is to be open and honest with your organisation and to encourage a learning culture by reporting adverse incidents that lead to harm, as well as near misses.

NHS Resolution (2017) states 'Saying sorry is:

- always the right thing to do;
- not an admission of liability;
- acknowledges that something could have gone better, the first step to learning from what happened and preventing it recurring'.

7.2.2 Support Your Team

At some point, almost everyone will have been a part of a complaint or an incident investigation. Can you remember how you felt when you were told? For the majority of those involved, it is one of the worst moments of their careers. They will often feel guilty, upset and anxious, not just about what may happen to them, but often about the outcome for the patient. Supporting staff through this process is important and can be the difference between a positive or negative outcome. It is important for the person you are supporting to know that as humans, we all make mistakes, it is how we learn from them and develop from them that is important.

It is important to explain to the person involved to remember that complaints or incident investigations are not formal, disciplinary or performance management processes; they are informal and designed to help us learn and improve our services.

Individuals who are the subjects of a complaint or incident investigation need to feel that they are fully supported by their manager. To be able to do this objectively, it is important to remember the following:

- Do not take sides during an investigation, either with the patient or the healthcare professional
- Reassure the individual that you are not interested in blaming anyone and you just want to find out if there is anything that can be done to improve the situation
- Do ask for advice if the situation is a particularly difficult one.

Keeping the person involved in the incident or complaint informed throughout the process helps to alleviate large amounts of stress. It is important that throughout the entire process, the individual's confidentiality is upheld and respected. They should see the final complaint response letter or incident report before it is distributed to those who need to be aware of the incident. It would be unfair not to let them see this and to have the chance to correct any inaccuracies. Reassure all staff that they will not be personally identified in any incident report.

Complex complaints and incidents can also feel daunting to you as the manager, so do not feel that you have to handle a difficult complaint or incident by yourself. Complaint managers are usually very experienced in most types of complaint and will be able to advise you further. The risk manager will also be able to help with any incident investigation, and any serious incidents will have a dedicated manager to help you collate evidence. If you feel you need more professional support, then it is important to look to your managers. This could be a matron, divisional nurse director or your director of nursing who, in many organisations, also has executive responsibility for clinical governance and quality. All of these will have experience in handling complex complaints and incidents or will be able to signpost you to appropriate support.

7.2.3 Know When to Stop an Incident or Complaint Investigation

7.2.3.1 Discovery of Significant Issues/Serious Failures

All complaints are risk assessed on arrival at your complaints department. If the risk is assessed as very serious, it should be referred to a more senior manager and a root cause analysis investigation will have to be undertaken. This means that your role would probably be as part of the investigation team and someone else will have responsibility for the overall complaint response. The complaints that you receive should be those that have been assessed as low or medium in terms of seriousness. The same goes for incident investigations. They will all be graded, and any serious incidents requiring investigation (SIRIs) will be handed over to a more senior manager for investigation.

However, if you discover during the course of your investigation that there are significant issues regarding standards, safeguarding or denial of rights, or serious issues such as grossly substandard care causing serious harm, you must refer it to your line manager for consideration of a separate investigation process (NMC, 2015).

7.2.3.2 When Disciplinary Action May Be Necessary

As previously mentioned, the complaints and incident procedures are entirely different from performance management and disciplinary procedures and must always be kept separate. You must stop the complaint or incident investigation process if you suspect any of the following:

- Professional misconduct
- Negligence
- Criminal activity

If you feel disciplinary action may be required, then you must alert your line manager. A formal investigation into the matter can then be arranged.

The patient or relative involved in the complaint or incident will be informed about what is happening and that you will not be continuing with the process until you have the outcome of the alternative investigation. Never do this on your own. It requires the authority of someone more senior within your organisation. If the individual's involvement only forms one aspect of a complaint or incident, you should be able to continue to investigate the other aspects, but you cannot do both investigations at the same time. Incident and complaint investigations are informal in that they are not punitive. The disciplinary process is very formal, and it is important the individual is advised to contact their union and/or professional body for support/representation.

7.3 INVESTIGATE COMPLAINTS APPROPRIATELY

The main aim of the NHS complaints procedures across the United Kingdom is to achieve 'local resolution'. This means that complainants should have their verbal or written complaint dealt with locally by the organisation which was treating them. If not satisfied with the written response, the complainant can be progressed to a second, more formal, stage. There are different procedures for the second stage depending on where in the United Kingdom the problem arose. It usually involves either asking for an 'independent review' or going straight to the Health Service Ombudsman.

This section focuses only on 'local resolution' because it is this part of the complaints process which involves the ward manager. It consists of either a verbal response to a verbal complaint or a written response to a verbal or written complaint. It may also consist of a meeting with the complainant followed by a letter.

7.3.1 Verbal Complaints

Wherever possible, verbal complaints should be dealt with immediately. A record of the conversation should include:

- the date and time,
- who was present,
- what information was given,
- any apologies made,
- any action that was taken at the time or future action you promised to undertake.

If the complaint was resolved at the time or within one working day, it can be regarded as resolved and closed. It is a good idea to keep a record of any complaints of concerns on the unit so that these can be reflected on and to monitor any trends of complaints. Many hospital policies now state that *all* comments, concerns and complaints should be formally noted. If a verbal complaint has not been resolved within one day, then it should be dealt with using the same procedure as that of a written complaint. All written complaints must go through the complaints department. If any form of complaint is made, it is important to ensure that those making a complaint are aware of the patient advice and liaison service.

7.3.2 Written Complaints

All written complaints should be addressed to the chief executive or complaints manager, but often, they may be addressed to the ward or unit manager. If you receive one directly, you must forward it immediately to the complaints department, they will send an acknowledgement to the complainant and sort out various aspects such as permission to access the patient's notes for investigation. Once you have received a written complaint from the complaints department with a request to respond, the following four steps are recommended:

1. Check you understand exactly what the complaint is about and what the complainant expects from you. In many organisations, a member of staff in the complaints department will have called the complainant and done this for you already. They will agree on a plan with the complainant and forward it on to you; however, if you are not clear from the plan what they mean, call the complaints department to clarify or contact the complainant. Maintaining personal contact in the early stages will help ensure the complainant is confident that something is being done. It is positively encouraged through national policy to keep in contact with the complainant throughout the process.

2. Appoint and support a member of your team to help you investigate. This helps junior team members to help understand the complaint and investigation process.
3. Once you have sufficient information, write a response/report or organise a meeting with the complainant and follow up with a letter. Often, complaints departments will have a specific framework for you to adhere to; ensure you liaise with them to help make the process easier.
4. Discuss the complaint, and any learning/actions from the investigation process, with your team.

7.3.3 Appoint a Member of Your Team to Investigate

There is no reason why other members of the team (both junior and senior) cannot be part of a complaints investigation with your support and guidance. It is good to be exposed to complaints early on in one's career. The fact that many complaints are due to poor communication and record-keeping will help your staff appreciate the importance of such matters.

For each complaint investigation, make sure enough time and support have been allocated. If necessary, go through the roster to ensure blocks of time can be freed up to carry out a thorough investigation. Work with your junior colleagues when speaking to individuals involved; it is important for them to be exposed to the complaints procedure and to understand how to approach staff when information is needed. This will help to develop them to be able to complete this part of the procedure independently.

7.3.4 Collate the Written Information

The investigation begins with the collation of relevant written documentation and meetings with the staff involved. This usually includes the following documents:

- The complainant's health records.
- Any trust-wide or local policies/procedures relevant to the complaint.
- Copies of relevant rosters or on-call rotas to identify who was on duty at the time.
- A copy of the original complaint and any other correspondence.

Relevant papers from the medical records may include medical and/or nursing progress sheets, consent forms, test request forms, GP referral letters, etc. Remember that physiotherapists and occupational therapists tend to keep separate case notes stored in their own departments and these may need to be located too. It is essential that you keep accurate notes of the investigation process in the form of a running log of events and findings. An example of an investigation progress sheet that could be used is outlined in Appendix 7.1.

7.3.5 Maintain Confidentiality

The complaints department will have informed the complainant that their records may be used and will have given them the option of refusing to allow this.

The Data Protection Act 2018 and the General Data Protection Regulation (GDPR) 2018 require all processing of data to be 'fair and lawful' and all 'personal data to be protected against unauthorised or unlawful processing and against accidental loss, destruction or damage'. This means that while the investigator has the documents, be they written or electronic, in their possession but are not using them directly, they should be kept in a locked drawer/filing cabinet and the office should be locked at all times when no one is there. Medical records should never be taken home under any circumstances; this includes any electronic records.

As a healthcare professional, the investigator should follow their own professional code of confidentiality and the Caldicott principles (Box 7.1). You should also ensure they are aware of the appropriate NHS Code of Confidentiality which emphasises that patient information must remain confidential and seen only by those with direct involvement (Department of Health, 2016).

In addition, remember to ensure that any information about the complaint, including the original letter, is not filed in the medical or nursing notes; it must be kept separately. This also applies to verbal complaints; no notes of any complaints should be filed in patients' records.

7.3.6 Interview Staff Sensitively

Once all the documents have been obtained, the next stage is to identify the staff involved and make appointments to see them all. Remember that this is not a disciplinary process; the purpose of the meeting is simply to ascertain the facts. Formal statements are not required; however, it is wise for the investigator to write some notes of the meeting simply to remember the facts.

If the complaint is complex, you may decide to ask for witness statements; in this case, you must ensure that the individuals are informed of their rights to

---

BOX 7.1 Caldicott Principles

1. Justify the purpose.
2. Do not use patient-identifiable information unless it is absolutely necessary.
3. Use the minimum necessary patient-identifiable information.
4. Access to patient-identifiable information should be on a strict need-to-know basis.
5. Everyone should be aware of their responsibilities.
6. Understand and comply with the law (Caldicott Committee, 1997).

have a union representative, colleague or friend present. You should also ensure they are aware that their statements may be used if the complainant decides to take legal action at a later stage.

The appropriate records should be made available when meeting with individual members of staff, to help 'jog' their memory. The staff member also has a right to see the original letter of complaint. If any members of staff involved cannot remember the patient or what happened, then they should say so; it is far better to admit this. In the final letter, you would simply say what you have concluded from the notes, but that the practitioner was unable to recall the details.

If at this stage you feel that the information cannot be assembled together within the time limit that was agreed, let the complaints department know. The complainant should also be contacted. You will need to explain what the problem is and say when you will be able to give a full response. Remember: always 'underpromise and overdeliver'. If you think you will get the information and response out within the next few days, give them a date for 2 weeks' time, this affords you some extra time to allow for unforeseen circumstances.

7.4 TIPS FOR CALLING OR MEETING WITH A COMPLAINANT

Simple complaints can often be settled with a phone call or a meeting with the patient, followed up with a written letter confirming what you have agreed. Inviting the complainant to meet and discuss the complaint can be a more successful option, particularly if they have lots of questions. Indeed, it is now encouraged as the first line of action on receipt of a written complaint. The complaints manager may or may not be involved, but it would be wise to use their expertise in such situations. Tips for holding a successful meeting follow.

7.4.1 Preparation

7.4.1.1 Arrange an Appropriate Venue

The meeting should be as informal as possible. It is preferable to use a non-clinical area, which is more familiar for the complainant. The complainant may bring other people with them for support, so it is wise to book a good sized meeting room that can accommodate several people. Make sure there are chairs available in a waiting area outside. If there are more than one member of staff involved in the complaint and they need to be present, it is best to call them in one at a time when needed. To be in the same room with a group of health professionals can be quite intimidating for most people who are not used to the clinical environment. The PALS provides confidential advice, information and support for patients, relatives and carers and can also be a source of support for patients and carers at this time.

7.4.1.2 Prepare a Draft Agenda With a Timetable

This does not need to be formal, but you will help to formulate a structure to follow, without, you may find yourself going around in circles on the same subject with no conclusion. A list of the complaints may be all that is needed so that you can go through each one in turn. It is also advisable to start by asking the complainant what they would like from the meeting. Often, those making the complaint will not have any experience of how a meeting with a healthcare professional should go, so they will often look to you to structure the meeting.

7.4.1.3 Try Not to Set Time Limits

For the complainant, this is their opportunity to go through a potentially traumatic experience. Telling them they only have an allotted amount of time could potentially produce a barrier before the conversation has even started. Although it is important not to set a time limit, it is important to be aware that a meeting of more than an hour will be taxing on both parties. If after an hour there is still no resolve, offer the complainant the opportunity to have a break, or if they would prefer, a further meeting to clarify any more details.

7.4.1.4 Make Sure That All Documents Are Available

Include case notes and copies of all correspondence pertaining to the complaint, as you may need to refer to these during your discussions. You may also wish to share the contents with the complainant so it is a good idea to familiarise yourself with the contents and be prepared to explain any words or phrases which they may not understand.

7.4.1.5 Ensure There Is Someone Else Present to Take Notes

These will be used to form the basis of the follow-up letter, so they will need to be detailed. If a nurse explained a procedure she undertook, for example, the notes would need to include that explanation. The more detailed the follow-up letter is, the more informed the recipient is. This also gives them something tangible to review if they forget the content of the meeting due to emotion or stress.

7.4.2 Facilitation

7.4.2.1 Listen Attentively

Make sure the complainants know they have your full attention. Turn the phone off and put up a 'Do not disturb' notice outside the door (including the date and time). If this is not possible, for example, you are an emergency bleep holder, explain to the family at the start of the conversation so that they are aware of your responsibilities. Ideally, if possible and clinically safe to do so, leave your bleep with a suitably qualified colleague. Make brief notes as you go and let them see what you are writing. One of the reasons you write notes would be to reassure the complainant that you are taking them seriously.

Show them that you are listening through body language and regular prompts. Summarise what they are telling you as you go along. This not only shows them that you hear what they are saying, it also ensures that you are clear about it in your mind. For example:

- 'Just to clarify my understanding…'
- 'Would you mind just going over that bit again with me?'
- 'I have the impression that you feel … Is that right?'
- 'If I understood you correctly, you have said…'

7.4.2.2 Empathise

Let them know you understand what they are feeling or what they must have gone through but ensure that you do not offer personal experience. For example:

- 'I can see why you must be upset'.
- 'It must have been difficult for you'.
- 'I can understand why you felt so angry at the time'.

Do not suggest that what they are saying cannot be true or insinuate that they must be exaggerating, with phrases like:

- 'I cannot believe she said it quite like that'.
- 'Are you sure that is what happened?'

This will only serve to aggravate the situation. It is advisable to neither agree nor disagree but remain neutral. Stick to empathising rather than sympathising, it will help focus the meeting on finding a solution rather than going through the problem over and over again.

7.4.2.3 Explain and Apologise If Appropriate

It is important to explain in non-jargon why things have apparently gone wrong. If there are nursing records pertaining to the situation, let them see what has been written and explain any technical terms that they may not understand. Be open; if it is clear that a mistake has been made, then apologise and be sincere in that apology.

The NMC (2018) notes patients expect to be told three things as part of an apology:

1. What happened
2. What can be done to deal with any harm caused
3. What will be done to prevent someone else being harmed

If there was no mistake, explain the situation surrounding the event they believed to have been incorrect. Often, something as simple as poor communication is the reason people feel mistakes have been made, so it is important to explain in a way they understand. Be aware that healthcare can be difficult for people to understand, so ensure they understand your explanation and consider rephrasing if they are still unsure. It will still be beneficial to apologise that they were not better informed and will ensure communication is highlighted as an action point from the meeting.

Make sure you have answered all their questions and allow time for further questions. Do not be afraid of silences. Good use of silence gives people time to think and feel that they are being respected and not rushed.

7.4.2.4 Agree on a Course of Action

Once you have listened, empathised and/or apologised and answered all their questions, you need to agree on a course of action:

- 'How would you like me to take this forward?'
- 'I suggest that from now on, we take the following steps to ensure it does not happen again … would you be happy with this?'

If the complainant is satisfied, ensure the course of action agreed is achievable. If what the complainant is asking for is not realistic, then say so. It would be unrealistic, for example, if you are asked to dismiss a member of staff for speaking to them in a cursory manner. In this case you might say 'I cannot authorise what you are asking for. This member of staff has been formally spoken to. I do not condone her actions but am prepared to work to improve her communication with close monitoring'.

Wrap up the meeting with a promise that you will look into things further if:

- what they are asking for is outside your remit;
- they begin asking for too much;
- they become angry and abusive;
- further issues arise at the meeting that you were not previously aware of.

A few well-chosen words are called for, for example, 'It appears that there are further matters that need looking into, so you will need to give me some more time to look into this properly'.

7.4.2.5 Close the Meeting Appropriately

Close the meeting by summarising what has taken place and what you have agreed. Always explain what will happen next, that a letter will be sent confirming what has been discussed with any changes that you have agreed to implement. Give a timetable; do not say they will receive a letter by the end of the week unless you are absolutely certain that you can get it done by then.

7.4.3 Follow-up

Always do what you agreed to do. If you have promised to call the next day once you have made further enquires, then do so. Even if you do not have the information, call and say so, then arrange to call again when you have the information. Follow-up is one of the most important stages in the complaints process.

Too many complaints reach the Health Service Ombudsman because complainants do not receive that call/letter which they were promised. Failing to follow up agreed actions only serves to make a bad situation worse.

7.4.4 Tips for Writing a Response Letter

7.4.4.1 Get the Structure Right

All letters should contain the following: a thank you (for raising the issue), an apology and/or a few words acknowledging the trouble it has caused them, an explanation of what happened, an outline of the action you are going to take, your contact details and an outline of what they can do next if still not satisfied.

If there are several subjects of complaint within one letter, prioritise the main complaint and address the minor points afterwards, using subheadings for complaints with more than one aspect of care helps to keep it structured. If you are unsure of how to structure a response, ask for support from the complaints department – they often have a structure to help guide people in their response.

7.4.4.2 Represent Your Organisation

Always keep in mind that your reply is representing your organisation and the overall healthcare system. Do not hide behind the system or processes that are beyond your own control; if the issue is beyond your direct control, say what your organisation is doing about it or who is trying to rectify the 'system problem'.

7.4.4.3 Write in 'the First Person'

Do not try to present an anonymous face. Refer to yourself as 'I' and the complainant as 'you'. For example:

- *Anonymous response*: 'It is worrying to hear that the standard of care was not satisfactory'.
- *Personal response*: 'I am sorry to hear that you were not satisfied with the standard of care'.

Addressing the complainant as 'you' signifies to them that you are treating them as a real person and not just another complainant. Try not to use the term 'we' unless you are explaining organisational policy or decisions. The complainant is much more likely to believe and trust a single person. An anonymised 'we' represents a faceless organisation.

7.4.4.4 Add the Personal Touch

It is always best to put yourself in the complainant's shoes and think how you would feel if you went through a similar situation. It is not just what you write, it is the way that you write it that makes the difference. The explanation and facts may be right but if they come across as formal and business-like, the complainant will not be satisfied.

Ensure your personality, professionalism and, above all, empathy shine through in the letter. The complainant will hopefully feel happy that everything that could be done is being done and that it is not just a standard bureaucratic response.

Another way to give your letter the personal touch is to write in the 'active' tense as opposed to the 'passive' tense. Consider the following:

- *Passive tense*: 'Please rest assured that action has been taken to rectify the situation'.
- *Active tense*: 'I can assure you that we are taking action to rectify the situation'.

The first sentence distances the writer and absolves any responsibility for the situation, whereas, in the second example, the complainant can be reassured that someone is making sure something is being done. Taking a passive and distant tone is more 'business-like' but not appropriate when writing to a complainant.

7.4.4.5 Avoid Using Jargon

Keep it simple or at least explain technical terms where you use them. Most patients do not know the detailed hierarchical structure in healthcare. So, using terms like healthcare support worker, physician, consultant, registrar or staff nurse should be avoided, or if you have to refer to these job titles then include an explanation about what they are. Try to stick to the generic terms 'doctor' or 'nurse'.

Use the same phrases you would use if you were talking to someone, not the official terms used in formal written communications. Use:

- 'about…' rather than 'with reference to…'
- 'I now know…' rather than 'I have since been informed…'
- 'because …' rather than 'due to the fact that…'
- 'I am sorry' rather than 'please accept my apologies'.

7.4.4.6 Start With a Thank You

First impressions count, so the way the letter starts is crucial; it sets the tone. This is why it is usually best to thank the complainant for the letter and for bringing the issue to your attention, followed by either an apology or a note of sympathy for their predicament. The opening paragraph should be kept short. Try not to use abbreviations such as 're:'. It depersonalises your reply immediately. Examples include:

- 'Thank for writing and bringing this issue to our attention'.
- 'Thank you for your letter about the problems you have had with…'

7.4.4.7 Apologise or Empathise

Follow your opening lines with an apology or a few words of sympathy. Remember that an apology is not an admission of liability within the complaints process (NHS Resolution, 2017). Empathising with the complainant does not equate to apologising. It shows that you are genuinely interested, supportive and understanding. Put yourself in their shoes and imagine how you would feel in the circumstances they describe. Show that you are making an effort to understand their point of view. If you have nothing to apologise for, then do not. You can say you understand without apologising, such as:

- 'It must have been frustrating to feel you were kept in the dark'.
- 'I can imagine this must have been very distressing for you'.

    If you are sorry, say so, even if it is just because the letter is late:

- 'I am sorry for the delay in replying'.
- 'I am so sorry to hear of your recent loss'.
- 'I am extremely sorry this has happened'.

7.4.4.8 Explain the Facts

Always give a full explanation of the facts but, again, make it personal. To say that 'this is what happened …' or 'these are the facts …' is too formal. Try the following examples:

- 'There seems to have been a major breakdown in communication in your case'.
- 'Unfortunately, it seems that the doctor forgot to tell the nurse he had prescribed the tablets to be given that night. The nurse had already given your father his tablets for the evening and so did not look at his chart again until the morning by which time it was too late'.

7.4.4.9 Outline What You Have Done or Are Going to Do

Outlining what you are going to do about the situation is the main part of the letter. The complainant needs to be reassured that something is going to be done as a result of their complaint. They need to know that their letter is being taken seriously.
    Here are some examples of how to begin this section:

- 'This has highlighted a gap in our system, so what I am going to do is…'
- 'As a direct result of your complaint, we have/will…'
- 'I can assure you that in order to reduce the risk of this happening again, I have decided to…'

7.4.4.10 Give Your Contact Details

Always finish by giving your contact details. A few extra words at this stage can help to make it feel more genuine. Here are some examples to stimulate your thoughts (and again to save you time):

- 'We will do everything possible to reduce the risk of this happening again'.
- 'Thank you again for bringing this to our attention'.
- 'I am sorry that we cannot be more helpful on this occasion, but hope you have been reassured that…'
- 'I hope this explains the position, but if you have any other queries, please feel free to contact me'.

Remember it does not take much to add the personal touch. Rather than write the usual 'please do not hesitate to contact me', the following will have a far better effect: 'I do hope this answers your questions, but should there be anything else you need to know I will be happy to discuss it further if you call me at... Alternatively, you can call our Patient Advice and Liaison Service at...'.

Giving them your direct contact details will hopefully ensure that any further issues can be solved through a telephone call.

7.4.4.11 Check the Layout Is Easy to Read

Once you have written the response letter, spend some time on making it look good and easier to read. Ensure the following:

- Use bullet points where you can to break up the text.
- Use subheadings if more than one complaint is incorporated.
- Have one idea per paragraph and keep sentences short.

7.4.4.12 Confirm the Final Letter (or Report) With All Staff Involved

The final letter or report must be checked and agreed by *all* staff involved in the complaint investigation to ensure it is factually correct. Confirm that all points raised in the initial letter have been answered, and the main one is answered first.

Once all those involved have agreed that it is a fair and accurate account of what actually happened, return your final response to the complaints department. Never send a response letter straight to the complainant. Most complaints procedures require that either the chief executive signs all response letters or a cover letter by the chief executive is included. The complaints team will ensure that this is done. They will also check through your letter to ensure it complies with various organisational procedures. For the more complex complaints (such as those involving other departments), you may only be required to send the results of your investigation to the complaints team and someone within the department will write the response from your report.

7.5 INVESTIGATE INCIDENTS APPROPRIATELY

Observe the trends from your incident forms and work closely with your team to reduce the risk of further incidents of the same nature happening again. Do not wait to be told what your main issues are from the risk management or clinical governance lead.

7.5.1 Incident Forms

Incident forms are an important part of any healthcare system. They empower staff to report not only mistakes but also external influences stopping them from providing the care they wish.

The purpose of incident reporting is to support you and the team to learn from incidents, understand trends and not place blame. Incident reports should concentrate on what happened and why, not who. The exceptions to this rule are:

- cases of gross negligence and
- if someone has been malicious, deliberately negligent or carried out a criminal act

Encourage team members to complete incident forms thoroughly and to think carefully about their responsibilities following an incident. Writing an incident form does not necessarily mean that the team member could not have found a local resolution themselves. In the section entitled 'Action taken', the team member can explain the initial actions taken to resolve the issue, e.g. a wrong infusion has been commenced on a patient and was stopped immediately when the error was found. The patient was observed and told at the time of the incident, and the unit coordinator and medical team were informed. This can then be reflected on when reviewing the incident – it shows that the team member took initiative to ensure that the patient was clinically safe and informed of the incident at the time. The team member successfully escalated their concerns appropriately and ensured that it was reported.

Copies of all incident forms are simply logged, and actions and responses are recorded. It is the role of your line manager or matron to ensure they are reviewed across the directorate on a regular basis to reduce the risk of further incidents. Take the initiative and do this first with your team; look at the trend of errors, is there a pattern? Are the same people involved? This gives you much more of a basis to improve patient safety by specifically targeting the problem areas.

7.5.2 Serious Incidents Requiring Investigation

If the incident constitutes a SIRI, your organisational policy will outline the steps you should follow regarding communications and dealing with the actual incident. A SIRI is an incident that:

- has resulted in serious harm or death;
- is of major public or media concern;
- involves allegations of abuse;
- threatens your organisation's ability to deliver healthcare;
- is one of the 'never events' (see Box 7.2).

If you are unsure, it is best to report it as a potential SIRI. A serious incident still warrants the completion of an incident form but, in addition, you should gather any relevant information, photocopy any relevant clinical notes, keep faulty equipment and gather information from witnesses within 24 h of the incident. This information will form the basis of further investigations. You should

---

BOX 7.2 The Never Events List

A 'never event' is a serious but preventable incident that should not occur with the appropriate systems in place. All 'never events' have to be reported both to the commissioners and the CQC in England and should be subject to a root cause analysis investigation (NHS Improvement, 2018).

Surgical

Wrong site surgery
Wrong implant/prosthesis
Retained foreign object post procedure

Medication

Mis-selection of a strong potassium solution
Administration of medication by the wrong route
Overdose of insulin due to abbreviations or incorrect device
Overdose of methotrexate for non-cancer treatment
Mis-selection of high strength midazolam during conscious sedation

Mental health

Failure to install functional collapsible shower or curtain rails

General

Falls from poorly restricted windows
Chest or neck entrapment in bed rails
Transfusion or transplantation of ABO-incompatible blood components or organs
Misplaced naso- or oro-gastric tubes

Scalding of Patients

Unintentional connection of a patient requiring oxygen to an air flowmeter.

---

ensure that your line manager is informed immediately as well as the senior teams involved in the patient's care. The patient and their relatives should also be informed but do not attempt to do this by yourself if you feel at all unsure. You should have specific training on communicating with patients and relatives following serious incidents.

An investigation team is usually nominated to undertake a further review in the case of confirmed SIRIs. You may be nominated to assist with the investigation and writing of the report. This is usually carried out using the root cause analysis approach.

7.5.3 Root Cause Analysis

The root cause analysis approach focuses on identifying the sequence of events and allowing the root cause of the incident to emerge. A serious incident is often not just the result of human error but a chain of events that led to the human error, so in that respect the term 'root cause' singular is often something of a misnomer as there is usually more than one 'cause'. The investigation should result in recommendations for improving systems and processes to prevent the risk of a similar human error(s) occurring again.

A senior person will be appointed to take the lead in the investigation and will gather a small team of individuals to assist. They will go through the following steps:

1. Data collection: this involves visiting the area where the incident took place, collecting information including the original incident report and any related policies, gathering statements and meeting witnesses.
2. Putting all the data in chronological order: some sort of timeline will be produced outlining what happened and when, and perhaps who was doing what at certain times.
3. Review meetings: a series of meetings will be held with the investigating team and any other relevant professionals (including those involved in the incident) to explore the data, using specific tools to help them pinpoint exactly what contributing factors led to the incident. The main contributing factors will then be explored in further depth to determine their root causes. A number of tools can be used; one commonly used tool is the 'five whys' (see Fig. 7.1).
4. Report: the lead investigator will put together a report detailing the investigative process, the identified root causes of the incident and recommendations for changes to be put in place to reduce the risk of further similar incidents.

If you or any of your staff were involved in the incident, you should be given the opportunity to review and agree the contents of the final report. Remember that this report is an analysis of the systems which were at fault, not the people involved. And like all reports, it should present the facts, not opinions, and demonstrate that the incident has been thoroughly and fairly investigated. It is not a tool with which to punish people. The whole point of incident investigations is to learn from them. If a mistake is made, it is usually an 'honest human error'. The only human errors that are punishable are those that can be defined as 'dishonest'.

If it is found during the investigation that a health professional has been dishonest in any way or has deliberately flouted protocols without any justification, then a different procedure will be used, usually the disciplinary policy. The individual concerned will be advised to contact their trade union representative; however, in the vast majority of cases, human error is caused by one or more system faults. It is absolutely wrong to discipline people for honest errors because it will only serve to stop us from being able to learn from the errors (Vincent, 2010).

There is a significant difference between a 'no blame' culture and a 'just culture' which is this:

All staff need to know

- If I come to work and intend to do something wrong – I am in trouble
- If I come to work impaired by drugs or alcohol – I am in trouble

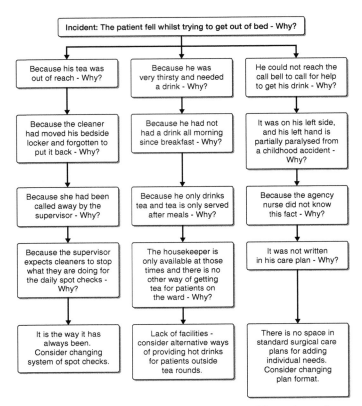

FIGURE 7.1 Five whys tool. An example of how it can be used for getting to the root cause of incidents.

- If I do something unsafe and I meant it (I was reckless) – I am in trouble
- If I do something unsafe and someone else could do the same, we need a systems solution

If you hear, or use, the phrase 'there but for the grace…', it is a sign of a system problem.

7.5.4 Contributing to Incident Investigation Reports

As a ward manager, you will probably not be required to write a full incident investigation report unless you have received full training and are appointed as a lead investigator; however, you may be asked to contribute some sections towards the overall report, so it is worth being aware of what is involved. There are lots of things to consider, for example, the patient or their relatives have the right to read the report, so you have to be sensitive to their feelings.

Incident investigation reports differ enormously from disciplinary investigation reports because they focus on system faults (that may or may not cause human error), whereas disciplinary reports focus on allegations of human misconduct or deliberate harm. This means that the staff involved should not be identified by name. Even the patient involved should be given a pseudonym, unless they and/or their relatives express a preference for their real name to be used. The report should also be written objectively in the third person. The NHS England (2015) Serious Incident Framework is a must read if you are ever involved in a SIRI or any other root cause analysis incident investigation.

When it comes to writing up the report the following headings are recommended:

- An executive summary.
- A description of the incident and its consequences.
- Pre-investigation risk assessment.
- Background and context of the incident.
- Terms of reference.
- The investigation team.
- The scope and level of the investigation.
- The investigation type, process and methods used.
- Involvement and support of the patient, relatives and carers.
- Involvement and support of staff involved in the incident.
- Information and evidence gathered.
- Chronology of events leading up to the incident.
- Detection of incident.
- Notable practice within the case.
- Care and service delivery problems.
- Contributory factors.
- Root causes.
- Lessons learnt.
- Recommendations.
- Arrangements for shared learning.
- Distribution list.
- Appendices.

Once an investigative incident report is finished you must ensure that you, and anyone else in your team who was involved in the incident, have the opportunity to read it and check for inaccuracies. Later, it is advisable to obtain a copy of the report for the rest of your team; this can be distributed via email or within the team meeting. This ensures that all learn from the incident, both from the recommendations and also by seeing first hand that incident investigation reports are all about learning and not punishing individuals involved. If any member of the team feels they need more support, or some clarification on the document, give them the time to sit and go through it together.

7.6 MAKE IMPROVEMENTS

7.6.1 Discuss Everything With Your Team

Discussing incidents and complaints regularly with your team is a good way of involving them in a collaborative response and resolution. It reduces the risk of staff saying, 'What's the use of filling in all these incident forms if no one ever reads them or does anything about them?' If you are willing to make improvements in practice, particularly as a result of incident reports, your staff will feel more encouraged to report them. The more incidents that are reported, the safer your working practices will be. The more you discuss patient complaints, the less your staff will feel threatened by complaint investigations and more open to learning from them.

Complaints provide you with important information and feedback about the experiences of patients on your ward. Incident reporting provides you with important information on safety issues. You must ensure that lessons are learnt from both. Make them a regular item on your team meeting agenda.

7.6.2 Follow Up With Action

Follow up all the actions at each meeting to ensure the issues raised previously are not overshadowed by the newer ones. A continuous plan of action from complaints and incidents should be maintained and updated regularly. This will ensure your team view them as an opportunity to improve services and make changes, rather than as a hassle.

7.6.3 Disseminate the Learning

7.6.3.1 Notice Board Displaying the Learning From Complaints

Getting no complaints at all does not mean you have a better service; it probably means the patients either do not know how to complain, are worried that you might take offence or that their future care may be affected. It is important that you state in your ward leaflet or information board that you welcome comments as a way of finding out what your patients really think.

Having a comment card system on your ward with a notice board for staff, patients and their relatives displaying 'You said, we did' is beneficial to everyone. It helps reduce the number of complaints but enables you to continue getting feedback. Without continuous comments and complaints, you can never be sure that the service you provide is truly meeting the patients' needs. You can put up extracts of written complaints (anonymised) and associated responses so that other patients and users of the service can see that you listen to their concerns and are actually doing something about it.

7.6.3.2 Notice Board Displaying the Learning From Incidents

This board is probably best displayed in your staff room. Like the comments/complaints notice board, it would be good to display the outcome of incident investigations but, more importantly, the actions that you have agreed to take with the team. The problem with running a department, 24 h a day, 7 days a week is that you cannot have all the team present at your team meetings. Displaying the results of your regular reviews and agreed action plans on a staff notice board will again encourage staff to be more open when reporting incidents and encouraged to see that they are being heard (and not punished).

7.6.3.3 Other Wards and Departments

Try to ensure that you are discussing the complaints and incidents across both your directorate and your organisation. Keep your matron informed so that they in turn can discuss the issues raised with their colleagues. You may be progressive in investigating and learning from complaints and incidents, but that will not necessarily be the case for all areas. Do not let it put you off sharing your practice with others, and thus hopefully stimulating them to share their practice with you too.

7.6.3.4 Action Points

- Ensure you are familiar with the origin of all quality indicators so that you can understand their significance and prioritise if necessary.
- Ensure that you and your staff receive appropriate training and support in handling complaints and incidents according to your local policy.
- If there is anything you are unsure about, get help early on from your line manager, complaints manager or risk manager. Better still, incorporate the complaints and risk managers into your network before you have to call on their services.
- Make sure the complaints or incident investigation process is halted if you suspect negligence, misconduct, a crime has been committed or anything that you feel requires a formal managerial investigation.
- If you do not have one already, put up an information board in your ward with comment cards and extracts of comments (anonymised) with responses, and an incident information board in your staff office.
- Inform and involve your team in all complaint and incident investigations and resulting action plans, preferably by having it on the agenda of all regular team meetings.

APPENDIX 7.1 EXAMPLE OF PROGRESS SHEET FOR A COMPLAINT INVESTIGATION

Action	Date Completed and Any Comments
1. Complaint letter received	
2. Contact complainant to clarify their expectations or any unclear issues	
3. Appoint member of team (if appropriate)	

Action	Date Completed and Any Comments

4. Meet with appointed member of team:
   a. Agree on issues to be investigated
   b. Agree on time out in diary to devote to investigation
5. Investigator:
   a. Locate patient's notes
   b. Find further relevant documents
   c. Identify and arrange to see staff involved
6. Investigator:
   a. Meet staff involved
   b. Find out what happened and why
7. Compile response letter or report
8. Check final response/report with all staff involved
9. Send final response/report to complaints department
10. Return patient notes to medical records department
11. Lock away the file in a safe and secure place

REFERENCES

Armstrong, D., 2010. The Power of Apology. Focus. NHS Education for Scotland.

Caldicott Committee, 1997. Report on the Review of Patient-identifiable Information. Department of Health, London.

Care Quality Commission, 2010. Essential Standards of Quality and Safety. Guidance about Compliance.

Data Protection Act, 2018. The Stationary Office, London.

Department of Health, 2016. TBC.

Francis, R., 2013. Report of the Mid Staffordshire NHS Foundation Trust Public Inquiry Executive Summary. The Stationary Office Ltd.

NHS England, 2015. Serious Incident Framework. NHS England, London.

NHS Improvement, 2018. Never Events List 2018. NHS Improvement, London.

National Patient Safety Agency, 2009. Being Open: Supporting Information: Patient Safety Alert NPSA/2009/PSA003.

NHS Resolution, 2017. Saying Sorry. NHSR, London.

Nursing and Midwifery Council, 2018. Duty of Candour. NMC, London.

Nursing and Midwifery Council, 2015. The Code: Professional Standards of Practice and Behavior for Nurses and Midwives.

Parliamentary and Health Service Ombudsman, 2010. Listening and Learning: The Ombudsman's Review of Complaint Handling by the NHS in England 2009–10. The Stationery Office, London.

Vincent, C., 2010. Patient Safety. Wiley-Blackwell, Sussex.

Chapter 8

Instigate a Rolling Recruitment Programme

If you could have all your vacancies filled at all times with the right staff with the right skills, would not life be so much easier? Unfortunately, this rarely seems to happen in real life, but you can go some way towards making things a lot easier for yourself if you concentrate on the recruitment process all the time, even when all your vacancies are filled. Nurses rarely stay in one post throughout their career. Change can be a good thing, however, and it is good for staff to regularly have new people join, with different skills to offer. It also helps you to continually review and change your staffing establishment according to the needs of your unit. Make sure you are always one step ahead so that when a person resigns you will be able to replace them quickly without causing too much disruption.

8.1 REVIEW THE POST WITH THE PERSON WHO IS LEAVING

Before you even begin thoughts of advertising and filling a forthcoming vacancy, you should first review the role with the person who is leaving.

8.1.1 Establish Why They Are Leaving

Staff may leave your team for promotion or to gain further experience. It could also be for personal reasons such as moving house, travelling or wanting to spend more time with children. You should be concerned if any members of staff are leaving for better working conditions, career prospects, better hours or because of any problems at work. Take note of why they are leaving and do something to ensure the next candidate will not feel the same way.

All members of staff have a right to fill in an anonymous exit questionnaire when they leave, but you need feedback too. You do not need them to fill in any forms; just ask them. Remember though that employees have the right to refuse an exit interview. They should always be voluntary and they can request a meeting with HR rather than you or your line manager.

When you ask why someone is leaving, aim to ensure the person talks a lot more than you do. Spend most of the time listening and taking notes (even if you do not agree). Ask questions such as the following:

1. Are there any other reasons for leaving?
2. What could we do/have done to persuade you to stay?
3. What have you enjoyed or found satisfying about working here?
4. What aspects of work did not you like or found difficult or frustrating?
5. Is there any more training and development you would have benefited from?
6. Is there anything that could be improved in the ward which would make things better from your point of view?
7. What is it about your next job that makes it more attractive than this one?

8.1.2 Establish if the Job Description Is Still Appropriate

Review the job description with them. Has it changed in any way? If the remit has grown to include other responsibilities such as a vital link nurse role, first ask any of your other staff if they would like to take it on. If not, consider adding it to the job description. If, for example, the person is a link nurse for diabetes and it is a much needed role on the ward, then think about recruiting someone who has, or is willing to develop, those skills. Add it to the job description before you advertise.

The job could have changed so much that the person leaving may say it needs someone more senior with specialist experience or perhaps even someone who does not need the skills of a registered nurse any more. If this is the case, review this idea with the rest of the team. You may all come to the decision that it would be beneficial to replace this person with someone requiring entirely different skills from another pay band. It is advisable in such cases to meet with your finance manager and line manager to go through what you would need to do to change the post and pay band but remain within budget.

8.1.2.1 Changing the Job and Associated Pay Band

You cannot change your budgeted 'establishment' immediately because it has to be done through the business planning process. However, you do not have to match the budgeted establishment exactly. You can recruit a Band 5 nurse into a healthcare assistant (HCA) post, for example, but only if you consult with your finance advisor and line manager first, to make sure that at the end of the year you will not go over budget in order to do so. The finance advisor will work it out for you, taking other issues into consideration such as:

- part-time staff in full-time posts,
- staff who are on maternity leave,
- staff on long-term sick leave,
- current use of agency and bank staff.

Try and think 'outside the box'. There is no reason why you cannot redesign the job into one that suits your ward. You may, for example, like to devise a new role such as an HCA who can also take on part-time ward receptionist duties. This could help enormously at times when your current ward receptionist is on annual leave or off sick. Likewise, if it is proving impossible to recruit Band 5 nurses, with your line manager's support you may look to create a Band 6 and HCA role within your existing budget allocation.

8.1.3 Review the Job Description and Person Specification

The job description may need completely rewriting or just a few minor changes. Do this together with the person who is leaving the job. Your HR advisor will advise you on what you can and cannot do with the job description according to your organisation's policies and procedures.

Redesigning roles when a member of staff leaves helps to replace outdated jobs and allows your remaining team to progress by taking on different responsibilities. You can design jobs around the patient and changing workloads rather than the other way around. It is not a difficult thing to do. The key is to ensure you involve the right people, i.e. your finance advisor, your HR advisor and your line manager.

8.1.4 Take Action if the Post Is Frozen or Removed

Unfortunately, it is not uncommon for ward managers to be prevented from replacing staff members when they leave. If your budget is cut back like this, then you need to take action to prevent the rest of your team from becoming overworked. Take some time to work out exactly what it will mean for your team. One less member of staff means that five shifts per week (i.e. 5 out of 21 shifts) will have one less person. You therefore have to make adjustments to your roster. Choose which shifts will have one less member of staff. For example, in order to maintain safety, you could cut one person from each weekend shift. However, you must not 'burn out' the rest of the staff working at weekends, so you would need to agree with your team which aspects of work will no longer get done at weekends. Patient safety and care are essential, so generally it could be the paperwork such as audits (performance indicators, etc.) that will not get done. Agree this with your managers – in writing. If they will not agree, then work together with them to identify something else (equivalent to the work of one member of staff per shift) that will not get done.

If you are already busy on every shift, then you cannot achieve the same amount of work with one less staff member. Find more efficient ways of working with the staff you have. Usually this means that you have to agree certain aspects of work will no longer get done or will get done in a different way. Do not just cope and allow your team to work extra unpaid hours to cover up for short-staffing. It contravenes the Health and Safety Executive (HSE) guidelines on managers' responsibility for balancing job demands with the availability of staff (HSE, 2011).

8.2 WRITE GOOD ADVERTS AND APPLICATION PACKAGES

Work with your HR department to develop adverts and application packages that will make your unit attractive to potential candidates. State exactly what you want in the advert and give them the material for your application packages. List what you want to be sent out to each prospective candidate.

8.2.1 Put in Extra Effort

Do not leave anything to chance. The recruitment teams in HR departments have a huge remit. They have to oversee the recruitment for all personnel within your organisation. They will send out standard application packages and do not usually have the capacity to make up specific ones for your ward. So, send them additional information to add to your application packages. If you really want to recruit the right staff, then you have to put in the effort, whether it is your job or not.

8.2.2 Writing the Advert

Involve your whole team in devising what to put in the job advert and include the person who is leaving as they are the ones who browse through the job adverts regularly. Ask them which adverts catch their attention and which parts of the job would be the most attractive for new staff. Getting that advert right is crucial. Most advertising is now carried out online through sites such as 'NHS Jobs' which means prospective candidates get to see only the first four lines of the advert at a glance, so concentrate on making these the most eye-catching.

Make the closing date for 3–4 weeks' time. If you give only 2 weeks, you are ruling out all potential candidates who are on annual leave at the time of the advert. Put the interview date on the advert too as it quickens the process. The interview date could then be around 2 weeks after the closing date. Having the interview date on the advert gives the candidate plenty of time to prepare. Waiting until you shortlist candidates before you decide on an interview date only serves to delay the process unnecessarily. You will also have a number of candidates who will not be able to attend, thus prolonging the process even further by having to set a second date. Make things easier and straightforward for you and the candidate by putting both the closing date and interview date on the advert in the first place.

Remember to attach the revised job description and person specification when you send the final advert to your HR recruitment department.

8.2.3 Application Packages

When the HR team receives enquiries, all they are required to do is send out a copy of the job description and person specification. Some send out information about your organisation too. If you really want to interest potential candidates, give your HR department further information about your ward.

Again, ask your team what they think would be good to include in the application package. A group of people are a lot more creative than one or two on their own. Possible options include:

- a photograph of your team, happy and smiling,
- a copy of your team's annual plan of goals/objectives,
- some quotes from your staff saying what is good about working on your ward,
- an explanation of your method of working, e.g. team or primary nursing, and perhaps even a sample of your roster showing how you organise yourselves and to prove that you do not expect them to work awful shift patterns.

Be careful not to give the impression that the ward is better than it is. The last thing you need is to recruit people under false pretences; they will not stay long. Disillusioned newcomers will disillusion your team.

8.3 SHORTLIST AND ARRANGE INTERVIEWS PROPERLY

Most healthcare organisations now have a database of professionals who have been removed from the register or any former employees or agency staff who should not be employed with you again. Before you shortlist the candidates, make sure that all the names have been checked against this database.

8.3.1 Tips for Shortlisting

1. *Shortlist within 5 days of the closing date.* Make sure you block out some time for this in your diary when you put in the advert.
2. *Shortlist with another person from your team.* Do not shortlist on your own. At least one of the people involved in the shortlisting needs to be on the interview panel.
3. *Base the shortlisting on the person specification.* Check that the candidates meet all the 'essential' criteria. The 'desirable' criteria need only be used when a particularly large number of candidates meet the 'essential' criteria.
4. *Keep a note of the reasons for selection and rejection of all candidates* which confirms that the same criteria were used for all candidates. Send a copy to the HR department, so that they can deal with any follow-up requests for information from rejected candidates. It will also help should there be any complaints or allegations of discrimination.
5. *Get the results of the shortlisting over to your recruitment department as soon as possible.* It is in your interests to show prospective candidates that this is a good place to work. Receiving an interview letter with only a few days to spare does not create a good impression.
6. *Try to ensure that requests for references are sent out at the shortlisting stage.* This will prevent any delays in offering the post to the successful candidate. Most application forms give the individual the option to not have references taken up until after the interview, so you need to make sure that you do not breach the individual's stated wishes.

8.3.2 Prepare for the Interviews

You will already have your interview date set from the advertising stage. You need a minimum of two people.

At least one of the interviewers should have had formal training in recruitment and selection, which includes information on the equal opportunity aspects of recruitment and the relevant legislation. Avoid having any more than three people on the interview panel as it can be intimidating to candidates at this level.

Holding interviews in your ward or department office is a good idea so long as you have the space and can guarantee there will be no interruptions. Make sure there is an allocated area outside the room where candidates can wait. The candidates will feel at ease because it is an environment they are used to. It can be daunting for clinical staff to enter formal office environments. They are unfamiliar places for healthcare professionals, particularly the more junior ones, and may serve to make them more nervous.

Remember also that there are obligations under the Single Equality Act 2010 to ensure that disabled applicants (or those that are carers or associated with someone who is disabled) are not discriminated against or disadvantaged in any way (see www.equalities.gov.uk). The HR team should have asked in the interview offer letter if individuals require any special assistance on that day. You should check before the interview if anyone has requested such assistance.

8.3.3 Prepare Your Team for the Interviews

Check the roster to ensure you have good 'numbers' on at the time of interviews and ensure all your staff are aware to be prepared for the arrival of prospective candidates. Agree with your team what they should do to greet them when they arrive. Everyone needs to create a good impression. Your staff on that shift should:

- keep a look out for the interviewees arriving,
- greet them warmly with a welcoming smile,
- show them where they can wait,
- inform them where the nearest toilets are,
- offer them a drink,
- offer to show them around the ward while they are waiting.

All this serves to confirm that your ward is a good one to work where all the staff are warm and friendly. Even if you do not offer the candidate a post, they will go away thinking what a nice place it is and tell all their friends and colleagues, who will tell their friends and colleagues. Word spreads quickly among healthcare staff. You do not want a disgruntled candidate telling everyone they would not have taken the job anyway because it did not look like a good place to work.

8.4 GET THE BEST OUT OF THE INTERVIEW PROCESS

Each candidate should leave feeling they have been welcomed, treated fairly and given every opportunity to demonstrate their suitability for the job.

8.4.1 Preparing the Questions

Prepare the interview questions in advance. Questions should be tailored to the person specification. In other words, you want to find out how the candidate meets the desirable criteria. You have already determined the essential criteria from the application form. Questions should also be included to find out:

- why they have applied for this job,
- what qualities they can bring to the team,
- their level of competence in practice,
- their awareness of wider nursing initiatives, such as Leading Change, Adding Value (NHS England, 2016).

You can also ask questions to get them to expand on what they have written on the application form. What you must never include are any questions about the candidates' personal circumstances such as how they organise their childcare or whether they are married or in a relationship.

8.4.1.1 Be Consistent

You should ask the same set of questions to each candidate. This is to ensure they all have the same opportunities to present the best of themselves. It does not mean you have to keep rigidly to the wording of each question. You can vary them according to the answers given. There is also nothing wrong with asking further probing questions to expand on the answer(s) given.

Try and stick to open questions to encourage the candidate to talk freely. The aim is to ensure the candidate does most of the talking. Avoid leading questions or closed questions. Encourage them to give their own answer, not the answer that you would like to be given.

8.4.2 Assessment of Practical Skills

It is very difficult to assess a candidate's practical competence in an interview. Presentations serve mainly to assess their presentation skills. One of the ways you can assess their practical skills is to include a set of questions based on scenarios:

- 'What action would you take if…?'
- 'How would you deal with a situation where…?'
- 'If X happened, what would you do?'

Another good way of eliciting information from candidates is to get them to quantify their experience, using questions like:

- 'How many times have you…?'
- 'What is your experience to date regarding…?'

The use of some sort of written test can help you to assess the practical aspects too. Present them with a couple of scenarios and ask them to write down what they would do. You could give them a situation where they have to prioritise as they would if they were in charge of a shift. Ask them to write down their rationale for each action.

If you decide to include a written assessment, you must do the following:

1. Let the HR department know at the shortlisting stage, so they can inform the candidates in the letter inviting them for interview.
2. Allow for the extra time required in the interview timetable.
3. Organise a separate quiet room where candidates can undertake the exercise undisturbed.
4. Make sure that the questions relate specifically to criteria outlined in the person specification.

Whatever method you use for assessment and interviewing, it is essential to set up a scoring system such as marks out of five for each question. Each interviewer will then score the person separately. These can assist with the final decision.

8.4.3 Prepare the Environment and Interviewers

Tidy up the room if needed. Set out the chairs, preferably so that you can see the clock on the wall behind the interviewee. Continuously looking at your wristwatch during the interview is disconcerting for the candidate. Sit in the candidate's chair to see if it is a comfortable distance away from the interviewers' chairs and there are no diversions such as glaring sunlight from the window.

Divert the phones and any pagers and ensure everyone turns off their mobile phones. Put a very big notice on the door saying 'Interviews in Progress' with the date and time. Include the time when you will be finishing.

8.4.4 The Role of the Chairperson in Interviews

Before you begin the interviews, identify which one of you will chair the process. Normally it would be you, but your junior staff members have to gain the experience some time and it is best they do it at a time when they can receive support and guidance from a more experienced interviewer. The role of the chair includes the following:

1. Introduce yourself and the other interviewers.
2. Settle the candidate by using small talk such as 'Did you find your way alright?'

3. Explain the interview plan and that you will be taking notes throughout the process.
4. Give some background information about your ward.
5. Facilitate the flow of questions.
6. Allow silences to ensure the candidates get a chance to consider their thoughts before answering.
7. Ensure that the candidate does most of the speaking.
8. Keep to the timeframe.
9. Ask if the candidate has any questions at the end.
10. Ensure they give you the appropriate documents, e.g. occupational health form, ID such as passport, etc. (HR will advise you beforehand as to what is required.)
11. Thank the candidate for attending.
12. Inform the candidate what will happen next, and when you will be making the decision.

8.5 FOLLOW-UP ALL CANDIDATES PERSONALLY

Make your choice and write up your notes immediately after interview. Keep all your notes and scoring results from the interviews. They help when feeding back to candidates, especially if you are required to feedback a few weeks or even months after the interview. Make sure the records are accurate and objective with no reference to personal opinions. Under data protection laws, candidates have a right to see these notes after the interview if they so wish.

Most people prefer to call the candidates personally. Do not promise to call them that evening. Remember: 'underpromise and overdeliver'. It will cause you undue hassle if you say you will call them that evening and then find that you are unable to make a final decision for some reason. Give yourself at least a day's grace, in case of any problems. Contact the person to whom the post is being offered first and work your way through the list of unsuccessful candidates. Always caveat any verbal offers stressing that the job offer will be subject to satisfactory checks, such as references and Disclosure and Barring Service clearance.

The references usually just confirm that you have made a good decision, but if they do not you will need to follow them up. That takes time. You can telephone the referees if you have not received a written reference. You can ask them to send you an email. A detailed record of the call including the date, time and the person you spoke to may suffice.

8.5.1 Calling Unsuccessful Candidates

Nobody likes to be the bearer of bad news. However, it is a nice gesture to call the unsuccessful candidates as soon as possible after the interviews, rather than let them wait for the official letter. Handle the situation by turning it into a positive experience:

1. Begin by telling the candidate they were unsuccessful.
2. Follow this immediately by telling them what they did well and which parts impressed you.
3. Then, tell them the reason why they did not get the job. Be precise but do not dwell on this part. Stick to one or two comments, then follow it up by offering further feedback at a later date should they want it.

Once the candidate is told that they have been unsuccessful, they are not usually in the mood to have a discussion about what they did wrong. However, they may want further feedback at a later date. Offer this service and make sure you are genuine in your offer. Tell them you have made lots of notes and are more than willing to spend time giving them further information about what they can do to improve next time. Remember that your aim is to make sure that everyone sees your ward in a positive light, even unsuccessful job applicants.

8.5.2 Follow-up Promising but Unsuccessful Candidates

If you only have one vacancy but two or three really good candidates, do not just take one and say goodbye to the rest. Speak to your colleagues. Do they have any vacancies? Does your HR team know of any other vacancies which you think the candidates may like to consider? Make a point of finding out this information before you call them. It is far better to let them know you think they have such good potential that you have talked to your colleagues and found another position they might like to apply for. Even if they are not interested, they will remain positive about themselves and have positive memories of the whole process.

8.5.3 Take Risks

If you know you have a similar vacancy coming up in another couple of months, consider taking the risk and employing one of the other good candidates as well. Obviously, you must get your finance advisor to work out all the costings and ensure you obtain your line manager's approval. It is usually a cost-effective way of dealing with things by the time you take into account the cost of further adverts and interviews.

8.6 ARRANGE A GOOD INDUCTION PROGRAMME

As soon as the candidate has confirmed their starting date, prepare their induction period together with your team. This is a crucial part of their employment. A good induction period makes the candidates feel welcome and reinforces their positive feelings about your ward. If you do not ensure this is done properly and then have problems later on with poor performance or incompetence, you could be found at fault because you failed to ensure an adequate induction period.

8.6.1 Before They Commence

You can start the induction before the candidate even starts the job by sending them any information that may be of interest together with a personal welcome letter from you. Include any forms that need signing to ensure they receive things in good time and save them unnecessary hassle, such as:

- car parking pass,
- email address and IT password,
- ID badge and security pass,
- uniform measurements.

Other items you might like to send them are:

- a copy of their 2-week initial induction programme,
- a copy of their first roster with details of shift times,
- a list of staff names in your team and any particular responsibilities, e.g. link nurse,
- minutes from the last team meeting,
- the name and details of their allocated mentor or preceptor.

8.6.2 Two-Week Supernumerary Period

It is advisable that the new recruit is supernumerary for the initial 2-week induction period (in addition to any formal organisational induction programme), making sure that they are not shown on the roster at all. If they are, there is the possibility that they may be used to cover in times of short-staffing. You cannot afford to let this happen in those first few weeks. Their initial induction should include the following:

1. *A warm welcome on their first day.* Make sure you or a senior member of your staff are there to greet them and can spend some time going through things with them.
2. *An induction checklist.* Most organisations have an induction checklist to be completed. Encourage them to complete this over the first couple of months, not the first 2 weeks. Do not overload them with information.
3. *Mandatory training.* Try and fit all their annual mandatory study requirements within the 2-week supernumerary period. If you get the statutory sessions such as manual handling awareness, health and safety and basic life support out the way in the induction period, it will not impinge on the study time available for the rest of your team in that financial year.
4. *Clinical work.* Allocate time for working full or half shifts during the induction period. They need to get the practical experience working alongside members of your team. Do not allocate them patients to look after on their own without support. That is not induction, it is using them as a pair of hands.

5. *Attendance at meetings.* Take them along to any meetings you have. Let them observe the ward managers meeting and perhaps even meet the director of nursing if present. Give them an insight into your role, vision and values right at the beginning no matter how junior their grade. It would be good to do this with all new HCAs too.

6. *Attendance to individual needs.* Tailor each induction programme to each individual. If someone has just returned to work after some time out, their needs will be very different from someone who has transferred from another department within the same organisation.

It is a good idea to develop the induction programme with someone in your team of the same grade as the new recruit. They will be more understanding of the individual's needs.

8.6.3 Allocate a Preceptor or Clinical Supervisor

Allocate them a preceptor or clinical supervisor and ensure this person is rostered to work with them regularly. Most areas will have some sort of competency package for new members of staff to guide their skill development during the first few months. If you do not, you should. Following this, they should have their first appraisal at around 3–6 months to agree objectives and a personal development plan for the coming year. Do not neglect this part; it is very important.

8.7 CONTINUALLY EXPLORE ALL OTHER AVENUES TO GET STAFF

You cannot afford to become complacent, even if you are 'up to establishment'. Always be on the lookout for new staff. If you create a warm and welcoming environment for anyone visiting your ward, you will hopefully end up with a queue of people wanting to work there.

8.7.1 Student Nurses

Word spreads quickly around student nurses about which wards are the best to work on, so make sure that all students allocated to your area are:

- warmly welcomed;
- addressed by their first name, rather than simply 'the student'. It matters;
- rostered to work with their mentor twice per week at the very least;
- given lots of feedback about their progress;
- invited to meetings.

If you do not receive students to your area because of your specialism, you will be losing out on a major source of future staff. Contact your local university and offer day- or week-long placements where students can shadow an experienced member of staff. Even spending a short time with you can make a huge impression.

8.7.2 Bank and Agency Staff

Some choose to work for the bank or agency on a permanent basis so that they can have more flexibility around their home life. However, they may change their minds and apply for a post on your ward if they see that they would have some choice over their shift patterns. In addition, make sure that your staff treat all bank and agency staff well by following ways:

1. Greeting them each time with a warm welcome and full introductions.
2. Taking time to find out the person's name, qualifications and experience.
3. Taking time to show them around the ward and going through their patients' needs with them.
4. Continually checking on how they are doing throughout the shift.
5. Giving feedback on how they are doing (temporary staff rarely receive this unless they have done something wrong).
6. Giving thanks at the end of the shift for anything specific that they have achieved or done well, not just general thanks for turning up.

8.7.3 Liaise Closely With Your Recruitment Lead

Most healthcare organisations employ someone who deals solely with nursing recruitment. Their job is to make sure everything is being done to attract staff to your organisation. They will have knowledge of all current recruitment initiatives such as the cadet nursing programmes, return to practice courses and various job fairs. They will have a good idea of what vacancies are where, plus who is interviewing for what and when. If you keep in close contact with your recruitment lead they can let you know of promising candidates from elsewhere. They will also keep you informed about when the next cohort of students is due to finish and start looking for jobs.

The recruitment lead soon gets to know which wards are popular and which are not. They will deter promising students from the worst wards where it is known they will receive little support and attention. They do not want to put all that effort into recruiting staff who would leave within a few months due to unsatisfactory working conditions.

You cannot blame the national shortage of nurses for all your vacancies. Nurses are out there and to find them you have to put more time and effort into:

1. making your ward one of the most popular wards to work on within your organisation and
2. finding the right places and right times to recruit.

8.8 DO NOT DISCRIMINATE

8.8.1 Part Time Does Not Mean Part Skilled

Nursing remains a female-dominated profession and, as a result, there will always be a high percentage of part-time workers. Healthcare professionals usually start off their careers working full time, but many will reduce to part time at some time during their careers in order to balance family and work commitments. This does not mean that they should be demoted or passed over for promotion. Do not assume that because a person does not want to work full time they are not as highly committed and motivated as those who do. If you do, you are being discriminatory.

In addition to this, some part-time workers will not apply for promotion because they have the impression that a higher-grade means working more hours. Try not to condone this culture; a higher grade means that higher skills are needed, not a higher number of hours.

If you do need to cover a certain number of shifts with a certain level of skill, then consider employing two people to share one job. Two people sharing one job will give you far more than one person in terms of experience. (You have to be careful that they are truly job sharing, i.e. not working the same shifts.) The key to this working successfully is to ensure they jointly take responsibility for the one role. In other words, they cannot blame the other for not getting things done.

8.8.2 Overseas Nurses Are Not All the Same

You may be familiar with the following expressions from nurses within organisations who have recruited from another country:

- 'They are all so hard working'.
- 'They do not understand that nursing is different here'.
- 'Where they come from, they do what the doctors tell them to'.
- 'They are quick to learn our ways'.
- 'They demand so much of our time'.
- 'They do not speak up'.

We would not dream of stereotyping all UK nurses in such a manner because we accept that they are all individuals. Yet people will often take the attitude that nurses who are trained in another country are all the same. Be careful not to condone this attitude. Accept that all these nurses are individuals, with their own unique blend of strengths and weaknesses. Work on their strengths as you would any other new member of staff.

Overseas recruitment is a fantastic opportunity to bring in new ideas and different experiences to your team as well as reflecting the diversity of the United Kingdom's population. It may be a hassle to ensure they have the appropriate competences and skills for the role but no more than any other staff nurse you recruit to your team. If you have a new recruit who is struggling in the role, look to improving your own systems of support and methods of staff development before blaming the individual nurse. If you undervalue individuals in any way, you will undermine their confidence and self-esteem. It will not help them work well. If you value each individual for the unique qualities that they bring to the team, they will feel good about themselves and consequently be motivated to work well.

8.9 SUCCESSION PLAN

8.9.1 Is Your Staffing Establishment Conducive to Good Succession Planning?

Think carefully about the mix of grades within your staffing establishment. If you only have one deputy, for example, you could be limiting promotion prospects for your staff. Having two deputy managers rather than one may be more helpful in terms of succession planning. If you have ten staff nurses and only one deputy, you may be putting yourself at risk of losing good staff who will look elsewhere to get in the next grade. It also reflects poorly on you if one of your senior staff leaves and you have nobody in your team who is ready to replace them. If this does happen, review and improve on what you are doing to develop the skills of your team.

8.10 FULLY INVOLVE YOUR TEAM IN ALL ASPECTS OF RECRUITMENT

People sometimes get the words 'inform' and 'involve' confused. Involving your team in the recruitment process entails more than just ensuring they are fully informed at each stage of the process. Keeping them fully informed is better than nothing but it will be far more beneficial to go one step further and actually involve them all in the process.

As soon as any team member resigns, meet your team to review the role and discuss whether it should remain the same or whether a different role would further enhance the team. Involve them in redesigning the job description if that is needed.

When you are ready to write the advert, get your team together to discuss and agree how to word the advert to make it more attractive to potential candidates. If you do not have time to meet with all your team, use other means of communication. Add it to the agenda of your regular team meetings rather than set up a special meeting.

8.10.1 Develop Their Interviewing Skills Early on

Include at least one of your team in the interviewing process. Guidelines usually recommend that at least one of the interviewers should be a higher grade than the candidate. There is no reason why you cannot include someone from your team who is the same or even a lower grade than that of the candidate; they have to start somewhere. Do not wait until staff nurses become a Band 6 before inviting them to sit in on interviews. The experience is extremely valuable. If they are only observing, give them one of the questions to ask. Everyone remembers their first interview when they had to ask questions and were too nervous to listen to the candidate's reply. It is something that should be done at an early stage in people's careers and not left until they are deputy or ward manager level (as is so often the case).

Take time after the interviews not only to discuss and agree the successful candidate but also to discuss the process. If you have a team member with you who is new to the process, ask what they have learnt. Discuss the process with the whole panel. Was there anything you felt you could have done better?

8.10.2 Get the Team Involved With the New Staff Member Early on

Once you have offered the post, let your team know who the new team member is and a bit about their background, then immediately appoint someone to take the lead in planning their induction. Make sure your culture of involving all the team also applies in turn to team members. In other words, encourage the person planning the induction to ask the rest of the team for their ideas on what should be included.

If you can, get someone of the same grade as the new team member to sort out the induction programme. They will understand the new person's needs better than anyone else. That includes HCAs; you do not need to be a registered nurse to be able to organise an induction programme for an HCA.

The key to having robust recruitment and retention is to ensure you show that you value the input from all your team members. It is the fundamental difference between leading your team and managing your team. Lead them well during the process and you will have a far stronger and healthier team than if you simply administer the recruitment process yourself.

8.11 ACTION POINTS

- Each time a member of your staff leaves, review the post and job description with the 'leaver' and the rest of your team.
- Involve your team in writing job adverts and customising the application packages for your ward.
- Include the interview date on all adverts and shortlist within 5 days of the closing date.
- Include your team in the whole process. Ensure at least one team member is included in the interview process and ensure all prospective candidates are given a warm welcome by your team when visiting the ward.
- Make sure all new team members receive a 2-week supernumerary induction programme devised by your staff and including mandatory updates.
- Network widely to ensure that you and your team are continually aware of new recruitment opportunities.
- Review your staffing establishment and systems of developing your staff to ensure they have every opportunity to develop the skills for the next post and are ready within 2–3 years of commencement in their current role.

- If you do not already do so, start involving your team in the whole process of recruitment rather than just keeping them informed.

REFERENCES

Health and Safety Executive, 2011. Management Standards for Work Related Stress – Demands. HSE, London.
NHS England, 2016. Leading Change, Adding Value: A Framework for Nursing, Midwifery and Care Staff. NHS, London.

Chapter 9

Be Politically Aware

Being politically aware is more than just understanding how central government policy affects the National Health Service (NHS). Political awareness is a broad area in nursing and can range from understanding an organisation's corporate structure, all the way to Westminster and understanding the current Health Secretary/Minister's agenda. Having this broad knowledge will help you to understand your role as a leader, better. It gives you a broader understanding on why decisions are made and the restrictions you may come up against. Political awareness, in the current climate of nursing has many facets, including the use of social media. This, to many, may seem like a small minefield to contend with, but it is simpler than most things, sometimes with huge rewards.

To be a leader and a manager, it is important that you have an understanding of the following:

- How your own organisation and other healthcare organisations operate.
- The health strategy and policy at a national and local level and how these may affect the service you provide.
- Who key people are (both internally and external to your organisation).
- How to use and embrace social media and understanding the positive impact it can have on your role as a leader (Hughes, 2018).
- The use of operational delivery networks within the NHS.
- External agencies that impact on nursing policy.

Building strong networks of likeminded nurses may also help to increase your knowledge base and help spread innovation throughout the field of healthcare. Learning to network and building alliances will help to build you as a strong and politically aware leader.

9.1 UNDERSTAND HOW HEALTHCARE IS MANAGED NATIONALLY

The NHS in the United Kingdom is made up of four NHS systems:

NHS England
NHS Wales
NHS Scotland
Health and Social Care Northern Ireland

Each of these individual services makes up the NHS as a whole. They are all funded by a taxation system, something that differentiates the UK health system from that of almost all other countries in the world in that it helps to ensure that care is free at the point of access to everyone and continues to be free to those eligible.

Each of the four countries has important differences in the way it spends its money in pursuing the goal of free healthcare for all. It is impossible to understand the multitude of intricacies each NHS service has, but it may help you understand your own service better by familiarising yourself with their structure, strategies and policies.

Having a simple understanding of these key areas may help benefit you in understanding why decisions are made at a local level to your own area of work. It may also give you a broader knowledge of the climate your own organisation is working within and why, sometimes, hard decisions are put in place.

9.1.1 The NHS in England

The Department of Health and Social Care (DHSC) is responsible for government policy on health and adult social care matters in England, along with a few elements of the same matters which are not otherwise devolved to the Scottish Government, Welsh Government or Northern Ireland Executive. It oversees the English NHS. Until 2017, health and social care were separate government departments, so this positive step means that both health and social care are viewed together. The DHSC sets out a yearly budget and a set of priorities, called the NHS Mandate, to set the direction NHSE needs to work towards and ensure that it is accountable to both the public and parliament. Mandates are usually multiyear documents to help NHSE plan long-term budgets and strategies to achieve the goals set. The work of the DHSC is supported by various bodies – these are known as agencies and partner organisations. These include the Care Quality Commission (CQC), National Institute for Health and Clinical Excellence (NICE), Public Health England (PHE), NHS Digital, Health Education England, Health Research Authority (HRA), NHS blood and Transplant (NHSBT), etc. At the time of writing (end of 2018) the regulatory body, NHS Improvement and NHS England were in process of merging as entities.

Clinical Commissioning Groups (CCGs) replaced Primary Care Trusts in 2013. CCGs are clinically led, statutory NHS groups that are responsible for the planning and commissioning of healthcare services in their area. They are responsible for 60% of the NHS budget and are led by a variety of healthcare professionals, including GPs, nurses, consultants, etc. The role of the CCG is vast and not only look at GP and hospital services in their area, they also look at the provision of all NHS service providers in their area.

In addition, the DHSC employs the Chief Nursing Officer (CNO) for England, who is the most senior nurse advisor to the government. The role of the CNO is to provide leadership to all nursing and midwifery staff across the healthcare system. Although they are the nursing advisor to the government, they do not advise on public health nursing which is a separate portfolio.

As a nurse leader, it is important to have an understanding of how the NHS structure works, including the work of your own local CCG. This will help you to have a better understanding of decisions made to your own services. If you are new to nursing management, the complexities of how the NHS is run, can feel overwhelming – accessing the DoHSC website can give you a broad overview to help with increasing your understanding.

9.1.2 The NHS in Wales, Scotland and Northern Ireland

NHSE is the most well known of all four NHS services; however, each country within the United Kingdom has their own NHS structure. These structures can often differ quite substantially from one another. Below is an overview of the differences between the structure of NHSE and the other three services.

9.1.3 Wales

In 2009, Wales underwent a large reorganisation of their services to help better equip them to deliver better healthcare to their changing landscape of healthcare.

Wales NHS services are commissioned by the Welsh Assembly Government, which produced the 'One Wales' strategy' document. This document looked at shifting hospital-based healthcare focus to public health and long-term care planning closer to peoples' homes. It focused on creating a 'wellness service' rather than a 'sickness service' by producing more joined up health and social care services. NHS Wales restructure in 2009 created single local health organisations that are responsible for delivering all healthcare services within a geographical area. This moved them away from the Trust and Local Health Board system that existed previously. Wales is now made up of seven local health boards and three Welsh NHS Trusts.

9.1.4 Scotland

NHS Health Scotland has a similar structure to that of Wales with 14 territorial NHS Boards, seven Special NHS Boards and one public health board. Similar to Wales, these boards are accountable to the Scottish health minister and the Scottish government health and social care directorates. The territorial NHS Boards are responsible for the protection and improvement of the population's health and delivery of frontline healthcare services. In 2010, the cabinet secretary for health and well-being developed a healthcare quality strategy for Scotland. This is the framework the NHS Boards work towards to ensure health goals for the population is met. In contrast to both England and Wales, Scotland and Northern Ireland also incorporate the provision of social services into the NHS Board directorate.

9.1.5 Northern Ireland

Similar to both Wales and Scotland, Health and Social Care Northern Ireland underwent a health and social care reform in 2009. This resulted in the formation of five health and social care boards, which are responsible for delivery of primary, secondary and community health.

Northern Ireland also has five regional trusts that cover the entirety of Northern Ireland. They also have five professional groups that form part of the executive agency responsible for the oversight, coordination and overall provision of health and social care.

Each country within the United Kingdom has its own CNO as their most senior nurse advisor to the government.

9.1.6 Private Healthcare

Private healthcare runs concurrently with NHS services. In England, private healthcare services must register with the CQC and thus meet the same care quality standards as the NHS. Many NHS hospitals now have their own private patient services, and the money generated in these units often help benefit NHS patient services.

There may be times as a ward manager, that private patients access NHS services within your own department. This may have some financial implications for you, as you can often reclaim costs of equipment and consumables, as well as time on the unit back. This is not something that you may come across on a regular basis; therefore, using your Trust's financial team to help with guidance is essential.

9.1.7 Be Aware of the Wider Organisation

Throughout our careers, we can be somewhat ignorant to how the NHS is run at a higher level. You are not alone; many of us would not have the need to understand the intricacies of the complex running of such a vast organisation. Our focus as ward managers is how we run our service, day to day. To have a better understanding of why you have to run your service in this manner, it helps to understand not just local, but national organisational structure. Once you become a nurse manager, you will find it helpful to become more aware of the structure and general running at both national and local level as this will also helps to give you a further understanding if you wish to progress up further in the managerial side of nursing.

All this information is now freely available on the relevant NHS websites (national or local).

9.2 THE VALUE OF THE BOARD OF DIRECTORS

In England, all NHS trusts have a board of directors, who are collectively accountable for the organisation. Every trust board is required to have a Chair and a mix of executive and non-executive directors.

Generally, the board comprises the following members:

- Chair × 1
- Chief executive × 1
- Executive directors × 5 (or more)
- Non-executive directors × 5 (or more)

9.2.1 Non-Executive Directors

Simply put, a non-executive director is a person who is a member of the board, but who has no responsibility for daily management or operations of the trust. The Chair of the board is a non-executive role. The Chair and non-executive directors are generally non-clinical people whose role is to provide good governance, give an independent voice, provide a level of scrutiny and make sure that the Trust Board is working in the interests of the local community. Many have business or financial skills, whereas others may have experience as a carer or even as a patient. The Chair and non-executive directors are not responsible for the operational management of the organisation. The idea is that they bring an independent and enquiring perspective to help the board to ensure a high-quality service. They are expected to draw from their experiences to make sure that the patients' interests are paramount.

Both the Chair and non-executive directors are employed part time on 4-year contracts. The Chair usually works 3 days per week and the non-executive directors work 2–5 days per month.

9.2.2 The Chair

The Chair's role is to lead the Trust board and ensure it fulfils all its responsibilities. The role entails chairing all the board meetings and ensuring the smooth running of the board by supporting, constructively challenging and setting the appropriate tone for the way the board works. The Chair's other key role is to communicate effectively both internally and externally to gain the views and commitment from the staff and the local community. This is why you will often see the Chair walking around the organisation with staff and attending various community and organisational events.

The Chair is part of a team that appoints the chief executive who then subsequently appoints the executive directors.

9.2.3 Executive Directors

Each executive director has a specified decision-making role and their ultimate goal is to design, develop and implement strategic plans for the organisation in a timely and cost-effective manner. Of the five executive director members, the following are a statutory requirement for all NHS trusts:

- Chief executive
- Director of finance

- Medical director
- Director of nursing and midwifery

The fifth executive director and any further appointments are at the discretion of the individual trust, for example, some appoint an executive director for human resources, others may decide on having an executive director for operations or planning.

In addition to the five executive directors, there may be a small number of further directors who are not in an executive role, such as strategy. This means that they attend board meetings and contribute to discussions and planning but do not have voting rights.

Executive directors are responsible for a particular function within the organisation such as nursing or finance, but as board members they are required to contribute to other trust-wide issues and policies outside their particular brief. All directors of the board have a corporate responsibility for:

- setting the strategic direction,
- ensuring effective financial planning and control,
- promoting quality and clinical governance,
- agreeing annual business plans.

9.2.4 The Chief Executive

The chief executive has personal responsibility for the overall operational management of the organisation and reports to the chairman. The chief executive is accountable for the trust's performance both in terms of meeting statutory requirements such as financial stability and health and safety legislation, as well as quality targets.

9.2.5 Getting to Know Your Board of Directors

The board of directors is a very powerful body and can often appear to be inaccessible to those not within the executive team. It can seem like a daunting prospect, especially those new to nursing management, to try and network with those within the executive team. There are many ways in which you can start to form networks with those on the board of directors, and not all of these require a face to face approach. We will look at the power of social media at a later stage in the chapter, but the use of professional social media platforms such as LinkedIn and Twitter can make directors more accessible.

The director of nursing is the nurse with the greatest authority within the organisation, they will be backed up by a senior nursing team, such as deputy director(s) of nursing, divisional nurses, matrons, etc. As ward managers, you will have frequent dealings with the senior nursing teams, and this will build your confidence in the structure and function of nursing management. Most people new to ward management may find it helpful to shadow senior nursing team members so they have an understanding of their role, and how they can support you in your role. This, however, is not only beneficial to those new to nursing management, anytime shadowing different roles will help to gain perspective of differing roles.

The board usually holds a meeting in public every month, which anyone can attend to listen and ask questions. Going along to these board meetings is a positive way of having an understanding of the issues currently facing the trust, and how they may ultimately impact you as a ward manager. Take junior staff along for the experience and to help develop their political awareness and understanding of organisational structure.

Many chief executives also hold regular 'open forums'. They book a couple of hours in their diaries where they will be available at a certain venue for anyone to come along and ask questions. These are not only information-giving meetings; they are there for the staff to raise and discuss any issues or concerns.

Another easy way of finding out what your trust board's priorities and plans are is via the intranet or in the annual business plan. This plan is open to the public and therefore written in an easily readable style.

It is useful to have an understanding of what the board's priorities for the trust are, this can ultimately help you set or adapt your own internal goals.

For those working in private healthcare, the system is less complex, but it is necessary that you make yourself aware of what your company's priorities are, if you have not already done so.

9.2.6 Board Meetings

The monthly meetings of the trust board can be extremely useful. It is worth putting the dates in your diary and if the pressures on the ward allow, try to attend to get an understanding of what is discussed and the format of a board meeting. Many junior staff often do not get the opportunity to attend board meetings even though they may wish to have a better understanding. Encourage your junior team to attend, either with you, or by themselves.

9.2.7 Ward Managers' Meetings

Most directors of nursing hold regular ward managers meetings in order to:

- find out what is going on at ward level,
- gain your views and opinions (which will influence decision-making at board level),
- discuss any issues that are currently affecting your practice,
- keep you informed about any changes in policies or guidance,
- get you involved in specific projects for improving patient care.

You will not be able to attend every time, so it would be constructive to make sure that at least two of your senior staff members are familiar with the meeting structure by inviting them to a meeting with you.

9.2.8 Directorate Meetings

Most NHS organisations are divided into directorates, divisions or business units. Meetings at this level are just as important for you to attend; however, as the ward manager, you may not always be invited to attend. Often, matrons and divisional nurse directors attend these meetings and feedback to ward manager level. There is nothing wrong with this approach; however, it may be worth asking your manager if they would help to facilitate your attendance to these meetings. Be willing to speak up in these types of meetings. You are on the frontline of nursing and understand the day to day running of your unit, use this experience to help with contributing to these meetings. Often, something that can seem small and insignificant in relation to the meeting may be a catalyst for a wider change.

9.2.9 Sending Staff to Meetings on Your Behalf

Sending other staff members to meetings on your behalf has multiple benefits. These not only include helping to reduce your workload but also show the trust and faith you have in your team.

Sending staff to meetings can be a scary prospect for some staff members; therefore, it is important to send members of staff to meetings with prior experience. Offer them the opportunity to shadow you at the meetings you wish for them to attend and be proactive in introducing them to regular attendees. This helps to give your staff member confidence as well as them having a familiar face in an often-intimidating room.

9.3 NETWORK – GET TO KNOW THE RIGHT PEOPLE

Networking has drastically changed in recent years. No longer do we need to be at large conferences to meet other likeminded people, we can now network with an array of people through social media. This will be looked at in more detail at the end of the chapter.

Networking, however, does not just mean making connections with influential people or even people within the same field as yourself. It is important to network with majority of people you will meet, from internal colleagues, such as porters, cleaners, personal assistants, to external colleagues such as charities, other trusts and patient advisory groups. Each person you network with will bring a unique set of skills and knowledge that you may be able to benefit from. The right people to network with are not always the most senior, and it is important to remember this on your day to day encounters.

9.3.1 Other Ward Managers

You should also cultivate a good friendship with your peers, whether this is other ward managers, or your own team of ward managers. Working in isolation from the managers of other wards and departments can have a negative impact when you may need to work together. Get together with the others as a group and you will strengthen your position and voice whilst also developing support and help for one another in times of pressure.

9.3.2 Senior Managers and Directors

Everyone in senior management will have had some experience of where you are in your management journey. Keeping this at the back of your mind will help to see them in a less intimidating manner. It is important to build relationships with senior managers and directors that are based on honesty, trust and integrity. Building these types of relationships help to ensure that when you may not agree with them, you are able to have an honest and constructive conversation with professional respect for one another. One way to build these relationships is to introduce yourself and your role and use the opportunity to reflect on the meeting in which you have both participated. Usually after such a meeting, the clinical staff dash back to their familiar clinical environment, but it is worth staying behind for a short while. Tidy up the coffee cups or put the chairs back in order to stop you feeling awkward. You may find you are drawn into a conversation with a senior manager asking you for your opinion about something from a clinical perspective. The more you do this, the more you will become confident in speaking with them.

9.3.3 Be Alert to Opportunities

Take your time to develop your network, it will not happen overnight. Utilising people you may already know to help with introductions can help with expanding your network that can then lead on to further connections. With the use of social media, this has become even easier to connect with people, and share ideas and innovations with one another. Having the appropriate networks can help to develop you as both a person and professional.

9.3.4 Building up Your Networks

Building professional networks of like-minded people whose main goal is to inspire and elevate one another will help develop you both personally and professionally.

Networking is based on mutual input from one another. There will be times where one person may be able to give more into the relationship due to circumstance or knowledge base, but this does not make it a one-way relationship. You may have something to offer that you may not even be aware of. Have confidence in your abilities and your successes and failures to help build effective relationships.

There are many ways to help increase your networks, and often, they are things you will already be doing subconsciously:

- *Helping others out.* Offer to send some information about something you have talked about and ensure you follow it up. Nobody forgets a simple, friendly gesture like this. Make sure you add your contact details on your cover note.
- *Saying thank you.* If you hear an interesting speaker at a meeting or teaching session, go up afterwards and thank the speaker. People rarely do this but speakers do appreciate feedback. This may or may not spark up a short conversation, which you could follow up afterwards. Whatever the outcome, they will remember you.
- *Social media.* The use of professional networks has reached beyond attending conferences or meeting people in person. The use of social media will be covered later in the chapter.

The simplest form of networking is to remember to be kind to all those you meet, offer whatever help you can, and do not be afraid to be honest. Remember that the junior staff you come across such as medical and nursing students may well get to be in more senior and influential positions than you one day. Try to ensure that they always remember you in a positive light.

9.4 BE DIPLOMATIC

9.4.1 Guard Your Opinions

Opinions are an important part of being a leader and a manager, but it is important to understand when it is best to share your opinion. If you are asked for your opinion, be constructive in your answers, making sure they are as factually based as possible. It is important not to bring too many personal feelings when formulating an opinion. Looking at the information presented to you and analyzing that is the most productive way of offering an opinion. You may also wish to refrain from offering an opinion, and this is also the right judgment call to make sometimes. Going away and reflecting on information before formulating an opinion also gives you time to critically analyse information given to you if you are unsure as to what is the best answer.

When you are asked for your thoughts or judgments, avoid using phrases such as 'in my opinion'. It would be better to present your opinion as a solution. For example:

Question: 'What do you think about the changes in the admission procedure?'

Answer 1: 'Well, in my opinion, the paperwork takes too long to complete'.

Answer 2: 'The paperwork could certainly be reviewed. It takes too long to complete'.

The second answer sounds like a well-considered answer, the person is confident and appears to know what they are talking about. Opinions are more likely to be accepted if presented as a fact rather than as an opinion, if they are presented in a confident and adept manner.

9.4.2 Avoid Being Unduly Critical

If you have problems with a colleague or a senior manager, it is important to not criticise them personally. Instead, keep a factual log of the issues you may be facing. This can then be reflected on without emotion, giving you a more unbiased account of the issues and helping to keep to professional standards.

9.4.3 Avoid Taking Sides

It is important to not take sides in times of conflict between others, as soon as you do this; you become part of the dispute. Stay objective and impartial, remaining calm and not being drawn in to the conflict. Calming down situations of conflict also gets you noticed in a positive light, in the same way, getting into heated arguments would be deemed as unprofessional.

9.4.4 Control Your Temper

You are only human, and you will have moments when your tolerance may be pushed, but it is imperative that you control your temper. Take a step back from the situation, even removing yourself from the situation all together, until you are calm and able to look at the situation in a rational light. Getting cross to a large extent is a choice and just because someone is angry at you does obligate you to get angry back. Literally, draw a few breaths and respond, do not react.

For example, if a major decision has been made without your consultation, try to not instantly react. Always think very carefully before you act and take time to analyse the situation. There may be a valid reason as to why you may not have been consulted. This does not mean that you are not within your rights to ask for an explanation but take the time to construct your response over the course of a few days, rather than producing a knee jerk reaction. Never respond to an email when you are cross. If you do want to do so, email yourself to your personal address and reread both the originator's and your response. Almost always you will be pleased you did not pressed send in the heat of the moment!

Usually there is nothing you can do other than accept a bad decision but take action to ensure something similar never happens again. Always learn from your experiences. It is usually best to let the individual(s) know how you feel about the decision but then leave it at that.

9.4.5 Think as a Manager

When problems occur, it is easy to see things from your own point of view, but it is the manager's role to regard things from the team and organisational perspective.

Consider things from a managerial point of view:

- 'How can I ensure adequate senior cover at weekends?'
- 'Will this pilot project improve patient care?'
- 'How will this benefit the staff?'

It is important to remember that whilst thinking as a manager, you still have an appreciation of the feelings your team may have. Communication is vital to ensure that everyone feels fully informed of situations that may impact on them.

9.4.6 Represent Your Organisation

An organisation is ultimately a team, all who have the same goal, directly and indirectly, of making sure that patients get the best care possible. There are instances, however, when things do not always go right, when internal struggle can impact on patients. Representing an organisation means that when things do go wrong, even if it is a specific department's failing, you represent the organisation as one of its managers. This ultimately means that if a patient complains about a particular service, even it has nothing to do with your own department, as a manager and a leader, it is important to empathise and reassure them that you will take their concerns forward to the relevant department, but that you apologise as an organisation. Likewise, when you are at a conference or other event, you are representing your organisation and your attitudes, behaviour and tone will be construed as reflecting the culture of the organisation for good or ill.

9.4.7 Voicing Your Disagreements

It is absolutely ok to disagree with something, what is important is how you put your point of view across.

You may wish to say, for example, 'If we are going to open up four more beds, we need to consider how it will affect the team' instead of, 'I think you are mad to even suggest it'. There will always be disagreements with others within your organisation but ensuring a professional level-headed approach to a resolution will mean that your concerns will be taken more seriously.

9.4.8 Understanding the Director of Nursing Role

The Director of nursing is the professional lead for nurses and midwives throughout the organisation and has a variety of lead roles within the nursing and midwifery workforce. They work closely with the chief executive and other board directors in making decisions about what happens in the organisation overall. A deputy/assistant director of nursing, who helps to ensure the key duties are carried out when the director of nursing is not available, often supports them.

9.4.9 The Professional Development Team

The director of nursing is responsible for the professional development of the nursing workforce and will usually have a small team of senior nurses to assist them in this role. This includes one or more deputy directors and various practice development nurses. It is wise to develop close working relationships with the deputy director(s) and practice development team. Their role is to help you and your team develop practice, so you should make maximum use of this resource. Much of their work is currently driven by national and local policy so close liaison will help keep you abreast of new policies and procedures.

9.4.10 Shadowing

Arrange to spend a day shadowing your nursing director if you can, to give you an insight into the role and responsibilities. If you feel too awkward approaching them out of the blue, introduce the idea via an email, explaining that you would like to learn more about their role and to pick up insights about how you can manage your ward more effectively. Many directors welcome this approach as it also gives them a chance to get to know more about what is happening at a clinical level in your area. They will let you know what dates they have available which will be appropriate for your learning.

9.5 GET RECOGNITION FOR YOURS AND YOUR TEAMS WORK

Often, celebrating successes within the NHS can be pushed to the back of most people's agendas. Getting yours and your team's success recognised and celebrated throughout the trust is important for staff morale as well as the potential of spreading innovation.

If you are unsure as to how to get recognition for you and your team's work, speak with corporate communications who will happily guide you.

9.5.1 Hospital Magazine/Intranet

Push yourself to do something you may have never done and write a small article for the hospitals magazine or intranet. It can be nerve wracking to do, but corporate communications will help to guide you as to how to write an article. It is also an opportunity to get junior team members to write about a particular innovation they may have been involved with or put forward ideas that other wards may benefit from. It could be something like a successful change in your handover system. One of the board directors usually has to read through and approve the newsletter before it is finally distributed. Your team's contributions will not go unnoticed.

9.5.2 Conferences and Study Days

Encourage your staff to speak about their successes at local workshops and conferences. Encourage people throughout your team to push themselves to publish in nursing journals and to submit posters to conferences. A leader's success is largely down to your team's ability to succeed and thrive, and a good leader is one that supports and encourages. You can find out about these through your organisation's practice development team or through local clinical networks. Keep them informed and involved in all new initiatives on your ward, they will hopefully tell others of your good work and help promote it to others too.

9.6 CHOOSE YOUR MENTOR AND MENTEES WITH CARE

9.6.1 The Mentor Role

When you become a manager, it is wise to have a mentor who is a lot more senior than yourself. The role of a mentor is to provide advice, guidance, information and contacts to help you in your work. A good mentor can be invaluable because:

- they have experience in your new field,
- they have often 'been there and done it' before,
- they will help you benefit from the knowledge they have in their current position,
- they can introduce you to their wider networks.

9.6.2 Choose a Mentor Who Is Right for You

You do not necessarily have to aim as high as possible to find the best mentor. If you are new to a ward manager role, you may find a long-standing peer who has done the job for many years will likely be more appropriate than a director of nursing.

This does not mean that at a later time in your own development, you cannot look for a new mentor to develop you.

Once you have found your grounding and want to look at moving ahead with your development, a member of the board is an ideal option to help. A non-executive director in particular can give you the benefits of their skills from outside the NHS, they are usually keen to take on the mentor role because they want to understand your role better. Having a mentee at clinical level gives them a valuable insight into the complexities of running a ward.

Your mentor may be able to explain how to get certain things done. If you feel you need extra staff for your unit and are getting nowhere, having a finance manager as your mentor can be extremely advantageous. Do not expect them to do things for you; it is not that easy. However, you can get them to explain the system clearly to you and point out where you could make changes to help facilitate your goal.

9.6.3 Change Your Mentor as Necessary

You do not have to keep the same mentor all the time. Set a limited time span such as 6–8 months to start with. By this time, you will have got to know them well and can choose to either stay with them or move on.

9.6.4 Your Team Are All Your Mentees

As a manager and a leader, shaping your team's future is important. Building on their key strengths and helping to improve their weaknesses not only helps to develop the person, but also the team as a whole. At one time, people would say 'do not waste time on people who are only looking to improve career prospects'. This advice is shortsighted and ultimately detrimental to your team and ward. Developing your team, even if it is with a view to move on to another job, has a more positive impact than not spending the time developing team members. Not only does this improve your reputation as a ward, but it also improves your reputation as an individual manager. Leadership is helping to lift people up and encourage them to strive for their goals. Some of the best team members you will come across will most likely be the quietest, so it is important to be aware of those who may not have a loud voice and help them to build their confidence.

9.7 PLAN AHEAD FOR YOUR OWN NEEDS

Being politically aware can also help you with where you want to go. Have you thought about where you are heading? You may wish to go into management, education, research or a more senior specialist clinical role (e.g. nurse consultant). Even if you want to stay where you are until retirement, it is still wise to plan ahead to ensure you get the best out of your job. The best way to do this is to review your own career development plan in your appraisal every 6 months. See if you are sticking to the goals you have set for yourself, and if your goals have changed, take the time to update your own development plan. Appraisals and development plans are not yearly tasks; they are a fluid continual tool to enable you to get the most from your career.

9.7.1 Identify Your Specific Interests

If your ultimate aim is to become a nurse consultant, start specialising in your subject now. Become a member of the appropriate specialist association and ask the appropriate clinical nurse specialist or medical consultant to become your mentor.

If your aim is to go into senior management, research or teaching, you would benefit by developing your skills in a particular area. Make sure that your name is linked with the specialist interest throughout the organisation. You could join the appropriate project group or perhaps even write an article for one of the mainstream nursing journals. Get yourself recognised and do not leave it to chance. That ideal job will not just fall in your lap; you have to make it happen.

It is easy to allow your own needs to get overlooked when your time is taken up with meeting the needs of your patients and staff. Boosting your individual status is something nurses find hard to do. You have to make your mark, so you stand out and your potential is noticed. Having a specific area of interest will enable you to do this. Although your job requires you to have a general knowledge of all issues, becoming an expert in one or two specific areas can help your future career prospects.

9.8 KEEP A FILE FOR YOUR CV

It is doubtful if anyone has the time or inclination to keep their CV up-to-date at all times, but it is helpful to keep a file (electronic or paper) and each time you attend a course, workshop or study session, add any relevant papers, certificates or reflective notes. You will find it easier when you come to writing your application, to have everything together in one place rather than having to search through papers and emails trying to remember what you did.

This has subsequently become easier since the introduction of revalidation by the nursing and midwifery council (NMC, 2015) by being asked to show your portfolio of continuous professional development every 3 years.

As well as the use of your NMC revalidation paper work, every job within the NHS is done so via NHS Jobs website. During the online application, the personal detail and statement are now your online CV for all jobs.

It is, however, still useful to have a paper CV to hand as part of your revalidation as well as presenting at interviews to give your assessors a physical copy of your skills and achievements.

9.8.1 Writing Your CV

The basic outline of a CV (see Appendix 9.1 for a sample CV) should contain the following:

- Your name
- Your address
- Your contact details
- A summary of your current role

Write a brief couple of paragraphs outlining your current role. This is one of the most important parts of your CV. Do not use the job description. Everyone knows the responsibilities of a ward manager. Promote what is special about you.

9.8.2 A Summary of Your Educational Achievements

List these in date order starting with the most recent courses. You do not need to include your school education; you are too senior for that to matter now. Your registered nurse qualification/degree should be the last one on the list.

9.8.3 A Summary of Your Work Experience

List your roles and the organisations where you have worked since registering as a nurse. Put these in date order starting with the most recent experience. Make sure to write in any key achievements you have, both professionally and personally. You need to celebrate what makes you unique, and how you can bring a new energy into a team.

9.8.4 References

Usually, two references are required, one from your current employer and one from your previous employer. If you have been in your current post for many years, you could use someone else like a link lecturer or course tutor. Remember always to ask your referees first. Never just assume that they will provide one as it is inconsiderate to put down someone's name as a reference without asking.

9.8.5 Tailor Your CV/Application Form to the Job

Each CV or application form should be tailored to the job you are applying for. Do not be tempted to include everything. No matter how senior or experienced you are, your CV should not be more than two pages long. Your potential employers need to see that you have the relevant skills for the job. They do not want to wade through everything you have done and have to try to decipher for themselves which bits are relevant.

9.9 POLITICAL AWARENESS AND SOCIAL MEDIA

Social media has become a huge part of everyone's lives, both personally and professionally. It had originally been seen as somewhat of a minefield to navigate as a professional, especially with the risk of bringing your profession into disrepute, potential of confidentiality breeches, as well as over stepping personal and professional boundaries.

Many organisations now actively seek to promote the use of social media to make the NHS and the work within it, more accessible to everyone. This can be right from the top of the NHS, including all the NHS organisations in the United Kingdom, to individuals' professional accounts.

Social media helps not only build individual reputations but also organisational reputation.

Each trust will have their own social media policy, most which will actively encourage their employees to engage with them by 'liking' 'retweeting' or 'sharing' posts.

There are many bonuses for the use of social media at an organisational level, these include:

- Building further awareness and reputations of the trusts
- Support local and national health campaigns

- Reach alternate audiences
- Improve service delivery
- Deliver fast and responsive incidents during major incidents
- Highlight good practice and celebrate staff success

Corporate trust social media is always run by the communications department. Many trusts now offer specific social media training to help highlight the risks and the huge benefits of social media within healthcare settings.

Advantages of using social media for individuals include:

- building and maintaining professional relationships;
- establishing or accessing nursing and midwifery support networks and being able to discuss specific issues, interests, research and clinical experiences with other healthcare professionals globally and
- being able to access resources for continuing professional development (CPD).

Guidance is now widely available from all professional registrations, including the NMC (2017), GMC and HCPC. Placing a copy of these in staff areas will help junior members of staff to understand their responsibilities when using social media.

It is important to ensure that your team understands that even if they are not using social media in a professional capacity, their personal social media accounts are held to the same professional standards. This includes patient confidentiality and bringing the profession into disrepute.

Engaging and encouraging junior members of staff to network via social media can be invaluable to the contacts they make. Many professionals now produce specific free education resources to help the dissemination of teaching and research – FoamEd (Free Open Access Meducation) being a good example.

9.9.1 Action Points

Access the appropriate websites each month to keep yourself up-to-date with what is going on nationally.

Find out the membership of your organisation's board and what their priorities are.

Aim to attend or send a representative to all the board meetings, sisters' meetings and local directorate/divisional meetings.

Aim to add at least one new contact to your network every few months.

Concentrate on presenting facts when asked your opinion and never criticise others.

Never use the phrase 'the management'.

Make a date to shadow your director of nursing.

Write a short article for your hospital's newsletter about a recent achievement in your ward or department.

Get yourself a senior mentor.

Consider whether your current mentees are relevant.

If you have not already done so, start a file (electronic or paper) for your CV/ next application form.

APPENDIX 9.1

Sample CV

Jane Smith
21 St James Street, Newbury, Gloucestershire GN23 4FN
Tel: 08900 400300
Email: jane.smith@internet.com.

Current role: Ward Manager, Flower Ward, Tree NHS Trust from 2008 to present, manage a 28-bed medical ward, using a primary nursing model, which I successfully implemented 4 years ago. I manage a team of 35 staff with a budget of £1.2 m. I use a bottom-up leadership approach in all aspects of my work by ensuring that I involve my team in all decisions and encouraging them to consistently challenge the status quo. I have a particular interest in the care of patients admitted with endocrine disorders and have developed a special interest group together with the diabetes specialist nurse on the care of patients with newly diagnosed diabetes.

Educational Achievements

December 2016: MSc in Health Service Management, University of London.

January 2010: BSc Professional Nursing Studies, University of London.

February 2007: RN, PgDip (PIN 123456 Exp 05/21), University of Surrey.

Career History

2015–present: Ward Manager (Band 7), Medical Assessment Unit, St Elsewhere, Manchester.

Key achievements: Decreased falls and infection rate by 60%. Reduced agency spend by 70% while reducing staff turnover to 8.5% and sickness to top decile against national benchmark.

2012–15 Senior Staff Nurse (Band 6), Stroke Unit, Another Trust, London.

Key achievements: Successful implementation of team nursing; instrumental in reducing staff vacancies from 50% on commencement of role to 10% vacancies within 1 year.

2009–2012 Staff Nurse (Band 5), 26-bed Medical/Endocrine Ward, Another Trust, Surrey.

Key achievements: Development of an in-house 1-year training programme to develop the skills of newly qualified nurses in caring for medical patients.

2007–2009 Staff Nurse (Band 5), 28-bed Medical/Respiratory Ward, Another Trust, Surrey.

Referees

Current Employer
Mrs A Smith
Medical Unit
St Elsewhere NHS Trust
016190 00000
jdeq@internet.com

Senior Lecturer
Mr B Jones
Faculty of Health and Social Care
University of London
08900 333333
jq@university.com

Case Study of Social Media and Impact on Patient Safety

#EndPJparalysis began life as a tweet by Brian Dolan in November 2016 and has since become a global social movement with >400 million impressions on Twitter. Its premise is very simple – to encourage patients to get up, dressed and moving while in hospital because of deconditioning, which is process of physiological change following a period of inactivity or bed rest that results in a decrease in muscle mass, weakness, functional decline and the inability to perform daily living activities.

As deconditioning something that can affect all ages and its solution is so simple, using humour, evidence, inclusiveness and building a strong sense of community which included Twitter chats, poems, www.facebook.com/groups/last1000days/, and a series of challenges such as the one million patient day campaign across the NHS in April to June 2018 and sponsored by the four CNOs of the United Kingdom, the spread was significant.

The results showed a reduction in length of stay, falls, pressure injuries and complaints as well as an improvement in staff well-being. The campaign has also spread to the Republic of Ireland, Canada, Australia and New Zealand and shares the classic features of social movements:

● They share a sense of **purpose**
● They are **united**
● They share **understanding**
● People **participate**
● They take **initiative**
● They **act**

At the heart of #EndPJparalysis is valuing patients' time as the most important currency in health and social care as it enables patients to get home sooner to loved ones. The simple question that you may wish to ask your own staff is this: 'If you had 1000 days left to live, how many would you choose to spend in hospital?' The beguiling simplicity of the question in which for most of us the answer would be 'Zero' means it can generate questions and ideas of how to value patients time and enable them to be discharged safely, sooner to loved ones.

REFERENCES

Hughes, K., 2018. The use of Twitter for continuing professional development within occupational therapy. Journal of Further and Higher Education. https://doi.org/10.1080/0309877X. 2018.1515900.

Nursing and Midwifery Council, 2017. Guidance on Using Social Media Responsibly. Nursing and Midwifery Council, London.

Nursing and Midwifery Council, 2015. Revalidation: How to Revalidate with the NMC. Requirements for Renewing Your Registration. Nursing and Midwifery Council, London.

Chapter 10

Look After Yourself

As nurses, we inherently want to care for others but are often terrible at putting our own well-being first. If we do not look after ourselves, and do not put our own well-being as a priority, how can we effectively look after those in our care?

Taking on a more senior role often brings a larger portion of stress, and often we put unrealistic expectations on ourselves. You may feel that you can never be off sick or that you feel you must be able to cope with any situation thrown at you. This, however, is not the case! You are only human, and just because you are now more senior does not mean that you will not be affected by things the same way.

We often hear of coping mechanisms, have you ever taken the time to think about what your coping mechanisms are, or if you even have any? If you have not, it may be a good idea to take some time to make a list of things that help you to cope with stressful or upsetting situations.

These may include the following:

- Exercise
- Spending time with friends and family
- A hobby
- Talking the problem through with someone
- Having some 'alone' time

Take the time to think about what helps your own well-being, but also remember that it is okay to not be okay!

When you were a more junior nurse, you will have felt that you had more support, that there was always someone more senior than yourself to turn to for knowledge and experience. When you become a ward manager, you become the person junior staff turn to for knowledgeable and experience. This change in role can lead to two issues–one of 'imposter syndrome' and another of worry about who you can turn to for support and guidance. Be safe in the knowledge that you are not alone, and you always have someone more senior to turn to for support and advice.

10.1 SET UP A PEER SUPPORT GROUP OR ACTION LEARNING SET

The ward manager's role is changing all the time. For some, you may be working alone; in others, there may be more than one unit manager. Whatever the setup of your unit or ward, remember, there is a whole plethora of support for you. Often, it can be difficult for ward managers from different areas to get together apart from if formal meetings are set. These colleagues, however, are often your best form of peer support as they will be performing a similar role and therefore have similar experiences.

There is no reason why you cannot set up a small support group of like-minded individuals. It's usually advisable to start off with a small number of around six people. Make sure your focus is on solutions and innovations to problems brought to the group. *Action learning* is a solution-orientated method of learning from each other's problems.

10.1.1 What Is Action Learning?

Action learning is a process that involves looking at problems from a different perspective, taking action and learning from the result of that action. The idea is that the whole group learns from the actions that the person takes rather than just one person alone. It involves a number of stages:

1. A member of the group presents their problem and the rest of the group listen without interruption.
2. The group encourages further reflection and discussion of the problem using an open and nonbiased questioning approach.
3. Following further discussion, the individual, together with the group, focuses on possible solutions. This enables the individual to devise a plan of action to tackle the problem.
4. After the meeting, the individual goes back to their workplace and follows through the agreed actions.
5. At the following meeting, the individual feeds back to the others what happened as a result of their actions. Together they discuss whether the action worked and what they learned from the process, i.e. if it happened again, what would they do next time?
6. If the action was not successful, another plan can be devised. The group can learn as much from unsuccessful approaches as they do from successful ones.

For further reading on the subject of action learning and how to get started, see Pedlar (2008).

10.1.2 Support and Challenge

Action learning is a simple but very effective method of learning and supporting each other. Ideally, it is good to begin with the help of an experienced facilitator, but it is not essential. If there is no one available within your organisation with the right skills and you do not have the funding for an external facilitator, do not let it stop you setting up some sort of 'peer support group' yourself. As long as you meet regularly, you will be able to help each other learn from your experiences and the actions you take.

The key to the success of your group depends on the following:

- Ensuring all discussions are solution orientated, as opposed to problem orientated.
- Meet regularly if possible.
- Ensure all discussions remain confidential within the confines of the group unless you agree the Chatham House rule (there's only one) that does not mean 'what is said in the room, stays in the room' – a common misconception. What you say can be shared, so long as the person sharing it does not directly or indirectly attribute it to you or your organisation.
- Sticking with the same group members as far as possible to enable you to build up trust in each other – but be open to welcoming new people into the group.
- Each member being voluntary, i.e. wanting to take part and actively contribute.

The group members need to be able to build up trust and confidence together to be able to challenge each other to think differently about things. Joint reflection with other ward managers is an ideal way of helping you become more effective in your role. It offers the chance to give and receive feedback from different perspectives.

10.2 DEVELOP THE ROLE OF YOUR DEPUTY

The deputy ward manager(s) can be among your greatest assets. Your aim should be to enable them to develop the skills and ability to do your job within 2 years of being in their current post.

10.2.1 'Acting Up' in Your Absence

When you take annual leave or if you are off on sick leave, you should be able to do so in the knowledge that your ward is in safe hands. You need to be confident that any issues that may arise while you are away can be dealt with successfully. The only way to do this is to prepare your team and to help them to develop the skills to 'act up' in your absence.

To prepare your team for this role, make sure that you share everything with them. They should be familiar with all aspects of your job. Take them along to meetings so that they are knowledgeable about the groups to which you belong and will be able to represent you in your absence. Do not ask them to replace you at a regular meeting when you have not familiarised them with the process beforehand; it would be unfair. They need to feel confident to speak up on your behalf. If you are just interested in getting the information, send your apologies. There is no need to waste your deputy's time. Read the minutes instead on your return.

10.2.2 Delegate to Improve Skills

Make sure your deputy has some exposure to the responsibility of your role such as parts of the budget, investigating complaints or writing reports on your behalf. Delegate early and support your team, teaching them process in a way they are able to undertake it independently; it is important that you do not just show them how to do it. Remind your team that even in your absence, there is still more senior support to turn to if they are unsure of what to do. Within the hospital setting, there is always a 24-h clinical site manager – they will be able to guide your team on any issues that arrive if they are unsure how to deal with it themselves.

Giving your team a broad understanding of the day-to-day running of the unit on a regularly basis helps to increase their confidence in standing in for you when you are away. Delegating tasks regularly will assist in their learning and development. If you do not know how to do something yourself, take the opportunity for you and your team to learn together.

Offering your team the chance to develop these skills not only gives them confidence but also gives more junior team members another person to approach when needing guidance.

10.2.3 Ensure They Get Appropriate Support

Make sure your deputy has access to a good senior mentor from elsewhere in the hospital. This will enable them to gain an external and thus more objective view on issues at work. A more experienced ward manager from another ward would make a good mentor for them. Your way is not always the only way, so having an external mentor will encourage them to get a different viewpoint and bring in extra ideas. This may not always be an available option, however. It may be helpful to send your more senior team members on coaching and leadership study days, whether these are in-house or external.

Encourage your deputy to join or set up a peer support group or action learning set. They also need an outlet in which to be able to discuss issues and learn from their experiences and mistakes in a safe environment with others who are in similar roles.

10.2.4 Work on Their Strengths

Your deputy will probably have strengths that differ from yours, so use this to your advantage.

When you undertake a managerial task in the presence of your deputy, such as dealing with aggressive relatives, discuss your performance afterwards. Identify together which aspects went well and which aspects could be improved. By doing this, you are enabling them to learn from your strengths. Do not feel threatened if your deputy picks things up quickly and performs better than you in certain tasks. Their skill in this area can give you the opportunity to delegate them the task and use the situation to your advantage. It will only serve to make your own job easier. Having a good deputy takes a huge weight off your own shoulders as it helps you to have peace of mind when you are away from the ward for any length of time.

10.3 GET YOURSELF A MENTOR

Having a mentor not only helps to achieve the objectives in your personal development plan but will also help in your day-to-day practice by giving you support and guidance or pointing you in the direction of someone who can help. It is advisable to find someone with the right position and experience to enable you to build your confidence in the role. If you are ambitious, a good mentor will also help you further your career.

Do not confuse a managerial mentor with the role of the mentor in nurse education. The role of the mentor in the world of management is totally different from the role of the mentor as advocated by health faculties.

10.3.1 Mentoring in Nurse Education

In nursing, the term mentor is used to denote the role of the nurse, midwife or specialist community public health nurse who facilitates learning and supervises and assesses students (both pre- and postregistration) in the practice setting (Nursing and Midwifery Council, 2008). Formal assessment and paperwork is associated with the role.

10.3.2 Mentoring in Management

Mentors for managers should be more experienced managers but *not* the individual's line manager. They usually meet regularly but do not work together in the same department. The relationship is more informal, and no formal records are required. It is a bit like clinical supervision except that the supervisor is an experienced manager rather than an experienced clinician. Managerial mentors may also introduce you to their networks so that you can broaden your horizons and become more politically aware.

Most senior managers within healthcare are familiar with the latter definition of the mentor role. Mentoring at managerial level is seen as a two-way process, in which it enables the senior managers to gain an insight into general issues at the clinical level. Like the clinical supervisor, the role of the mentor in management is to

- offer a different and objective view of the issues you wish to discuss;
- offer a nonjudgemental relationship;
- develop your skills of reflection to enable you to continually learn from your experiences;

- advise, guide, support and help you to solve problems;
- help widen your network to give you more of an insight into the politics of the wider organisation.

Do not choose a mentor because they are 'nice' or you happen to know them. Find someone who can help you reach the goals in your personal development plan. If, for example, you wish to develop your skills in dealing with patient complaints and writing response letters, the complaints manager or one of the nonexecutive directors who is involved with the complaints department would make an appropriate mentor. As mentioned previously, nonexecutive directors can make ideal mentors.

10.3.3 How to Approach Prospective Mentors

It is not easy to approach someone you do not know and ask them to be your mentor. One option is to shadow them first. Shadowing a senior experienced manager is now being widely encouraged by managers and trusts. If the day turns out well and you feel it would be beneficial, you can then ask them to be your mentor. Otherwise, thank them for their time and find someone else. Unfortunately, being able to do this during your working hours may be difficult and may only be able to be facilitated in your own time. Mentors are by no means mandatory but can offer you a support system.

10.4 CHOOSE YOUR SUPPORT SYSTEM CAREFULLY

10.4.1 Members of Your Team

Your team is very much your family when you are at work; you celebrate each other's successes and share in each other's failures. Although you will work together as a team and hopefully have some good times together, it is wise to not to use them as a sounding board for any work-related problems you face. If you are frustrated, angry or upset because of a situation at work, talk to your mentor, clinical supervisor or friends and families outside of work. It is important to understand that showing emotion is not a weakness, you are a human and showing emotion is part of being a good leader. If you are always seen to be stoic and devoid of emotion, it can make your team feel that you may not be as passionate as they are; however, do not let your emotion lead to accusations of unprofessionalism.

10.4.2 Your Line Manager

Be open and honest when talking to your line manager about your problems and frustrations. This helps to show the respect you have for your line manager. When discussing any problems or frustrations, go with potential solutions or with an idea of how you would like the problem to be resolved. By doing this, it gives your line manager an idea of ways they may be able to help you. Asking for help is not a weakness, and, just as you would like your staff to feel they could approach you when they were struggling, your line manager will be the same.

10.4.3 Be Wary of the Informal Network or Grapevine

You can never be sure who knows who, who is related to whom, and what sort of relationships people had before you joined the organisation. The director of nursing could have trained with your line manager and still meet socially. Your ward receptionist may happen to be a good friend and neighbour of the chief executive. The only safe bet is to ensure you never talk negatively about anyone or that you do not say something you would not be happy to say to them personally.

10.4.4 Get to Know Influential People

When you attend a work gathering such as a meeting, presentation or conference, try not to stick with your peers where you feel safe and comfortable. You already know them and see them regularly. See if there is anyone there that you could meet, perhaps someone who will introduce you to another part of your organisation. Try and make an effort to talk to someone that you do not already know at meetings.

10.4.5 Be Conscious of What You Say

If you speak in negative tones, the people you talk to will generally return those negative tones. If you use positive language, people will generally be positive in return. If you criticise others, you will be criticised. If you gossip about others, they will gossip about you. What you give out is what you will get back. Always consider the mnemonic **THINK** before you speak.

Is it **T**rue?
Is it **H**elpful?
Is it **I**nspiring?
Is it **N**ecessary?
Is it **K**ind?

Be careful also of those who try to manipulate you into divulging information, using statements such as 'I hear your line manager has been having problems with the team in ward X'. Never agree with a statement such as this. Reply with something like 'I know nothing of it' or 'Have you talked to her about what you've heard?' Never be drawn into such conversations even if you agree and do not like the way your manager is handling things. Let your manager know how you feel by all means, but never let it be known to others. Disloyalty earns disrespect.

10.5 REDUCE STRESS

Nursing staff through tradition and training are good at spending a great deal of mental, emotional and physical energy on caring for others. Taking time to think about caring for yourself can be daunting and difficult (RCN, 2017). Understanding stress, and the effect it can have not just on you, but your entire team, will help to develop good coping strategies.

Epel et al. (2018) state there is an almost unbounded set of human experiences that can fall under the umbrella of 'stress'. The term stress is frequently used in both scientific circles and colloquially to refer to a number of different processes that are related but distinctly different. For example, 'stress' is sometimes used to refer to actual life events or situations that happen to a person, such as losing a job or divorcing a spouse (hereafter 'stressors' or 'stressor exposures'). Stress is also used to refer to the cognitive, emotional and biological reactions that such situations evoke ('stress responses'). In other words, how you react to the *excessive pressure* or *other types of demand* determines the amount of stress you feel.

You will always have pressure of some sort or other in your work. A certain amount of pressure is needed to keep you motivated, and while we know about good stress and bad stress, if it exceeds your capacity to cope, it can make you ill. Stress is not just felt by you, but it is also collectively felt as a team. Stress risk assessments are a good tool to help understand the pressures faced by yourself and your team and can help with referrals to occupational health if it is starting to impact on your work or day-to-day life. When you are in the midst of dealing with continual excessive day-to-day demands, it can be difficult to recognise the signs. Ask yourself the following:

- Do you often think at the beginning of the shift 'here we go again'?
- Do you find there are more bad days than good days?
- Do you constantly feel that you cannot get things done, that the barriers are too big?
- Do you feel that you simply do not have the energy to do the job anymore?
- Do you find that you are always busy, doing too many jobs at once, trying to be available to everyone?
- Do you take increasing amounts of work home with you and/or does thinking about work keep you awake at night?
- Do you find it more difficult to switch off, even on your 'days off'?
- Do you increasingly suffer with continual aches and pains, a tight stomach or indigestion?
- Do you increasingly suffer from frequent colds and infections?
- Do you feel more anxious than you used to?

It is important to recognise the symptoms of stress. These are just a sample. If you allow them to persist, you are risking serious health problems. It is important to understand what triggers a negative stress response in you, and it would be advisable to speak with occupational health to help with workplace stress.

10.5.1 Coping With the Pressure

The job you are doing is inherently stressful; after all, you have an extremely responsible job. It is normal and healthy to feel stressed on some days, and you will have good and bad days. It is not normal when you are stressed every day and there are no more good days. If you do find things are just getting on top of you, then it is a good idea to stop and think if there are different ways of doing the job or ways of coping with its inherently stressful nature. These include the following:

1. Going to see your manager to identify and agree areas where your workload can be reduced.
2. Identifying areas for further training and development to enable you to deal with certain pressures.
3. Setting up a group with your peers to support and learn from each other's experiences.
4. Having a mentor or clinical supervisor to help you deal with difficult situations and learn from them.
5. Thinking about your own health and lifestyle.
6. Developing a robust amount of coping strategies.

10.5.2 Think About Your Own Lifestyle

You should also think about the way you are leading your life right now. We often forget about our own health and well-being in the pursuit of caring for others. Look at your current lifestyle. Do you have

- poor health habits (e.g. smoking, consuming too much alcohol, processed food and fizzy drinks, not getting sufficient exercise)?
- negative attitudes and feelings (e.g. dwelling on mistakes, thinking everyone else is right)?
- unrealistic expectations (e.g. expecting all staff to know everything and work as hard as you do)?
- perfectionism (e.g. expecting work to be completed to the same standard even when adequate staffing or resources are not available)?

How can you make these more positive? Work together as a team to develop better health and well-being practices not just for yourself but also for your entire team. Organise team events such as a race – this will give you all a common goal, you can support one another, and you could use it as a way of boosting charitable funds for the unit. Try not to isolate yourself from your team, being the unit manager does not mean that you have to exempt yourself from work social events; participate in workaway days, such as trips or dinners – these give you time to bond with your team and improve your own mental well-being. Technology can be helpful, too: Try out a few mindfulness apps or devices yourself and pass them on. Good apps include Calm, Headspace, and the Muse.

10.5.3 Look After Yours and Your Team's Health

You need to be in the best of health to be alert enough to make the right decisions and support your staff. Hospitals are hot, humid places and you are on your feet all day. If you do not drink water regularly throughout your shift, you will suffer from symptoms of dehydration. Staying hydrated can be difficult on busy shifts, but ensure staff are supported in rehydrating themselves. Make it possible for them to have water bottles in clinical areas. We would not let our patients go 12 h with no fluids, so why should we expect this of staff? Regular breaks are also essential to ensuring good health for all team members. Ensure the team works together to enable people to take adequate breaks, and if there is an increase in clinical demand, make yourself available to help clinically to support staff to be able to take a break. If you make time at work to eat and drink sufficiently, you will not only be more alert and productive at work, you may also have some energy left for when you get home. In addition, you are exposed to many varieties of viruses and bacteria at work, so need to ensure that you are in good physical health to prevent you succumbing to illness. Ensure that all staff are aware of how occupational health can support their well-being and encourage them to access these services if and when possible.

10.5.4 Take Time Off When You Are Ill

Going to work when you are not fit enough is defined as 'presenteeism' and is particularly widespread among those who work longer hours within the NHS. The Royal College of Physicians (2015) have noted that 68% of NHS staff in England and 70% of NHS staff in Wales report having recently attended work despite not feeling well enough to perform their duties.

It is used to be generally accepted that the body needs time to rest during illness and time to recuperate afterwards. In the past, if you were ill you took time off work to allow your body to 'fight' the illness, and an extra few days to ensure that you were fit enough for return. Nowadays it seems to be accepted that you should work through the illness. Hodgkinson (2005) illustrates this exceedingly well by describing the Lemsip adverts through the ages. These originally focused on the 'steaming cup of smooth nectar' that was 'part of the delicious and much-needed slowdown that illness can bring into our life'. Nowadays their adverts, like many others, focus on getting us through the day. Take a pill. 'No time to be ill. No time for bed. Go, go, go'.

If you are ill, your body needs time to recuperate. Your health is more important than your job. In addition, going to work with an infectious illness (i.e. a cold) really is not wise, particularly when you are infecting sick, vulnerable patients. Try and set an example for your staff. If you have a nasty cold or flu, stay at home and encourage the rest of the team do the same.

10.6 LEARN FROM MISTAKES AND EMBRACE THE EXPERIENCE

Success is the result of good judgement, good judgement is the result of experience, experience is often the result of bad judgement (Robbins, 2001).

Any nurse who says they have never made a mistake is lying. We are humans, and it is human nature to make mistakes. The key is to learn from them and do not dwell on things. In any job, you will make mistakes; it is all part of the learning process. It is so easy to feel pressured when you have made a mistake, particularly in the clinical environment where patient care may have been compromised. The worry over a poor clinical decision, the distress from having upset people or the anguish of feeling you have let the side down can be overwhelming, discuss with your line manager about the concerns you have. They can often provide reassurance and a debrief of the situation.

Try and deal with your mistakes in the following three stages:

1. Take corrective action and/or ask for help as appropriate.
2. Talk it through with someone (individual or group) and learn from it.
3. Take action to reduce the risk of you making the same mistake again.
4. Incident report the mistake.

The key is to be open and honest, never cover up, always talk it through with someone and learn from it. If you allow yourself to continually worry about your mistakes, it will increase your stress levels and gradually affect your health and self-esteem.

10.6.1 Be Wary of Perfectionism

Are you a perfectionist? Most of us like to think we are, having high levels of standards goes hand in hand with being a nurse. There is a difference, however, between high standards and being a perfectionist.

Perfectionists tend to get more upset when under pressure and are more likely to cover up mistakes than others, they are also less likely to ask for help. Excessive worry over mistakes puts perfectionists at risk of developing mood disorders and even phobias (Kawamura and Frost, 2004). If you have tendencies towards perfectionism or are a perpetual worrier, you need to work on changing your mindset. This is not always an easy thing to do, but with the right support, be it from your line manager or occupational health, you can reduce this level of stress drastically.

Discuss any mistakes with your peer support group and let others learn from the experience too. Experience is built on mistakes, and the most successful people you will meet will have failed at some point, often many times to get to where they are now. If you allow your mistake to make you think and feel negatively, you will become reluctant to try new things, treat mistakes as learning opportunities.

10.6.2 Be Confident

There will be times where you play the incident over and over in your head – this is a normal reaction, and you will often find yourself thinking, 'it's all my fault' or 'if only I hadn't done this or that'. This again is a normal reaction to making a mistake, whether you are the most senior member in the organisation, or the newest staff nurse – if you did not feel this way, this is more of a concern. What is important is ensuring that these incidents do not affect your confidence. Be honest and say something like 'Sorry about that. It was my decision and with hindsight I accept it was not appropriate. I guess the best thing to do now is …'. This helps to show you acknowledge your mistake and are looking for solutions to move forward. This is an example of good leadership; often junior staff feel that their seniors and managers never make any mistakes – this helps them to relate to you better and see that even the most experienced make mistakes, but it is how they move forward and keep their confidence that is the true lesson.

10.6.3 Dealing With Mistakes – Changing the Culture

Most healthcare policies and strategies are now focused on being open and honest; this has been further embedded in practice after the tragedies at Mid Staffordshire NHS Trust and the subsequent Francis report. A national reporting system was set up to record mistakes, adverse incidents and near misses and to make sure that lessons are learned, and people are not punished. The aim is to promote a blame-free culture, which encourages people in the health service to report mistakes without fear of reprimand. Changing the mindset of people working in the NHS after years of punishing people for mistakes is no easy task. There are still some healthcare managers who continue to perpetuate a 'blame culture'. Nurses today still may not feel entirely comfortable with sharing information when they have made an error, particularly one that has resulted in harm to a patient.

You can help by being a role model, show your staff that you learn from your mistakes and help them to discuss and learn from their errors. Create an environment where they can admit and learn from their mistakes without being under threat of punishment or blame. Remember that root cause analysis investigations should investigate the system(s) that led to the error, not the person(s). Do not ever allow it to be otherwise.

10.7 REMEMBER IT IS ONLY A JOB

Do not let yourself succumb to work-related burnout. You are at risk if you regularly

- work more than 37.5 h per week;
- take work home with you;
- come in on your 'days off' for meetings or to catch up with things;
- think about work when you are not there;

- allow staff to call you at home;
- cancel days off or annual leave because of work commitments.

If you are allowing any of the above to happen regularly, then you are investing too much in your job and not enough in other areas of your life. Take action now, it is your choice. Take stock and think about what you can do and what you will do to ensure that you lead a more balanced and fulfilling life rather than putting all your energies into work.

The first step is to try and prioritise your workload to fit into 37.5 h per week. The next step is to review what your priorities are outside of work. These could include getting exercise on a regular basis, seeing more of your family, spending evenings out with friends, taking up or renewing an old hobby. It is important that you find that balance.

Plan to take some annual leave every 3–4 months and book it at the beginning of the financial year. Do not save it up; spread it throughout the year to give yourself regular breaks. Avoid the 'if only' way of thinking:

- 'If only we had more staff …'
- 'If only I could get on top of all this paperwork …'
- 'If only the roster didn't take me so long …'

Do not prolong getting your life in balance by waiting for all the 'if only's'. You could be waiting a very long time! Do not let life pass you by, enjoy the journey not just the destination.

The reason why you are in your job should hopefully be because you gain job satisfaction. If you are not satisfied in your role, it is up to you to make some changes; if not, there is always the option of leaving and moving to a different job, even if you resort to doing some agency work for a time. Sometimes, a break serves to allow you to stand back and take a look at your life, think about what you enjoy and what you really want to do. Put yourself first, not your job.

10.7.1 Action Points

- Get a group of five or six other ward managers together and set up an action learning group to learn from each other.
- Focus on developing the skills of your deputy so they can fully support you in your role, especially in your absence.
- Think about getting yourself a mentor or clinical supervisor.
- If you are under too much pressure at work and feeling stressed, identify possible solutions and take action.
- Take steps to ensure that looking after your own health is a priority, including taking sick leave when you are not fit for work.
- Focus on learning from your mistakes rather than worrying about them.
- Ensure you have a competent and confident team behind you by encouraging staff to be open and learn from their own and each other's mistakes.
- Book some annual leave to take every 3–4 months. Work to live; do not live to work.

REFERENCES

Epel, E.S., Crosswell, A.D., Mayer, S.E., et al., 2018. More than a feeling: a unified view of stress measurement for population science. Frontiers in Neuroendocrinology 49, 146–169.

Hodgkinson, T., 2005. How to Be Idle. Penguin, London.

Kawamura, K., Frost, R.O., 2004. Self-concealment as a mediator in the relationship between perfectionism and psychological distress. Cognitive Therapy and Research 28, 183–191.

Nursing and Midwifery Council, 2008. Standards to Support Learning and Assessment in Practice. NMC, London.

Pedlar, M., 2008. Action Learning for Managers. Gower, Hampshire.

Robbins, A., 2001. Notes from a Friend. Pocket Books, London.

Royal College of Nursing, 2017. Stress and You: A Guide for Nursing Staff. RCN, London.

Royal College of Physicians, 2015. Work and Wellbeing in the NHS: Why Staff Health Matters to Patient Care. London, Royal College of Physicians.

Chapter 11

Be a Good Role Model

A good leader sets standards concerning the way their staff and patients should be treated. A major part of your role is to set an example for your staff to follow by showing them:

- how you expect them to conduct themselves;
- how you expect them to treat the patients.

Behaviour and attitude is highly contagious, the way you behave has a huge effect on how your team behave. If you encourage, support and feedback positively, it will have a positive effect on the rest of your team, hopefully creating a domino effect.

11.1 BE SMART

Where expression of feelings and attitudes are concerned, people are very much influenced by how you look and sound, a lot more than by what you say.

Appearance counts; there is no doubt about it. Just because you have a set uniform, it does not mean that you do not have to bother with what you look like. The image you present to others at work will be seen as a reflection of your level of confidence and self-esteem. The way you control your posture and use your body language can persuade others that you are more or less confident than you might actually be feeling that day.

11.1.1 Uniform Policy

Make a point of adhering to your organisation's uniform policy. It helps set a standard for the rest of the team, and if you are asking your team to adhere to something, you yourself must be the first to set the example.

It is important to help facilitate your staff to adhere to the uniform policy; even simple things can make a big difference. Do staff struggle when they are on a run of consecutive shifts, to have enough clean uniforms? If so, speak with your team member and see if acquiring them another uniform will help. Take the time to understand the reasons as to why they may not be adhering, and work together to ensure that they do.

11.1.2 Set the Standard With Your Own Uniform

1. Make sure your uniform is clean and stain-free.
2. Make sure your shoes are clean and/or polished. Many clinical areas have specific shoe policies – for example, theatre nurses may have to wear specific shoes for that area. Make sure that you are aware of what shoes are permitted in your area, to help guide your team as to what is appropriate for their clinical area.
3. Jewellery policies are often specific to each individual trust, but one common theme throughout is that staff, for infection prevention and control reasons, are bare below the elbow. Ensure that no watches or bracelets are worn. With regards to other jewellery, ensure that your team is aware of what is acceptable to wear within the policy. You can then advise them to not wear any other jewellery in to work, or provide them with secure lockable storage (such as lockers) to keep them in.
4. Ensure that you have a name badge, which displays your name and designation. Many trusts have now adopted the #hellomynameis campaign to highlight the importance of introducing yourself to patients. If your trust has not done so, it may be the opportunity to lead this change.
5. Most uniform policies, especially within clinical areas, state that staff should keep their hair off the collar and tidied back neatly and off their face. This is both practical and important for infection control.
6. Do not neglect your hands and nails. The majority of clinical areas do not allow false nails or painted nails – again, this is due to practical and infection control reasons. As clinicians, however, we are continuously washing our hands and using alcohol gel – all which can have a detrimental effect to yours and your staffs' skin. Ensure hand cream is available to staff, and refer to occupational health if any staff have issues with their skin.
7. If you are working in a nonclinical capacity and are not required to wear your uniform, it is important to remember you are still representing the organisation that you work for. Most trusts have a nonclinical uniform policy to help with any questions you may have.

11.2 MAKE A GOOD FIRST IMPRESSION

First impressions are powerful and permanent, and you never get a second chance to make a good first impression. People form an opinion within the first few seconds of meeting you, so it is important to get your image right with all new acquaintances. It is important to understand different types of body language and how they can impact a first impression. Folded or crossed arms across your torso is a very defensive position. Where possible keeping an open position, arms either side of you and smiling will put people at ease and help them to feel comfortable meeting you.

11.2.1 Visitors to the Ward

Show your staff the way you would like all visitors to be greeted. Everyone in your team should take the initiative in making people feel welcome. There will be times where staff are exceptionally busy and may not be able to welcome visitors as soon as they arrive. Guiding your team to acknowledge them, such as 'Hello, I will be with you as soon as I have finished…', means they can carry on their task uninterrupted, but visitors will feel as they have been acknowledged. Ensure all your staff wear proper name badges, with their name and designation clearly identified. The enormous array of uniforms and job titles in healthcare today make it extremely confusing for people to work out who is who and who does what. While they are not a substitute for a personal introduction, they do help visitors recognise who people are. Many wards and units now have a team board, with each staff members picture and name so that visitors can review and have an understanding of the different uniforms on the unit.

11.2.2 New Members of Staff

Make it your aim to greet all new members to the team; starting a new job is a daunting experience. Having someone come over, introduce themselves, shake your hand and ask how you are is a very welcoming experience and one that is often not forgotten. New junior doctors become future consultants and GPs. Student nurses may well go on to become future nurse managers with whom you will liaise. Those first impressions of being on your ward will stay with them.

11.2.3 Centre the Spotlight on the Other Person

The key to making a good first impression is to centre the spotlight on the other person. Demonstrate immediately that they are the centre of the conversation. This is particularly pertinent in the case of patients and their relatives. They are not there to hear about you; they want to feel confident that they have your full attention and that you are in control. Think how you would feel as a relative presented with the following greeting:

> 'Oh hello. We are a bit busy at the moment. I'm afraid that your father's admission was unexpected. We are a little short staffed, but I promise I will come over and see you as soon as I can'.

This greeting is focused on the person who is making it and creates the impression that they are not in control of things. If you focus your greeting on the other person, it creates a far better first impression:

> 'Hello there. Your father has been admitted to bed 10. If you'd like to take a seat in the dayroom, I'll come and explain everything to you in about 20 min once we've settled him in'.

It is important to ensure that visitors feel reassured that their relatives are in a safe and caring environment. It is important that, even when a new admission has made the dynamic of the ward more difficult, their relative is going to receive the best care possible.

The same applies when you are meeting other health professionals:

Focus on self: 'Hello. I'm the ward manager. I've been here for a good few years and know how the place runs like the back of my hand. If you need anything, let me know'.

Focus on other person: 'Hello. You must be Mark Smith. I understand you've just started, how are you settling in?'

While both greetings are perfectly acceptable, the latter example demonstrates that if you focus your greeting on the other person, it can help them to feel a lot more comfortable and relaxed. Using the name of a new acquaintance also makes it more personal.

Focus also on listening to what the other person has to say. You will make a good initial impression if you demonstrate good listening skills. Give positive verbal cues such as 'that's useful to know' or 'what happened next?' Try not to take over by giving unsolicited advice or relating a similar experience; this only serves to refocus the conversation on to you. Aim to listen to your new acquaintance, not to make them listen to you. It also helps if you maintain steady eye contact. Do not be constantly looking over their shoulder thinking about what you should be doing next. Try not to interrupt by answering the telephone or busying around doing other things.

Giving a good first impression gets you off to the right start and will save a lot of time and effort later on.

11.3 ALWAYS TRY TO SMILE AND BE POSITIVE

Your facial expressions affect the mood of your team. When you smile at someone, they will feel happier in an instant; few people would not smile back. It makes people warm to you. There may be times, when smiling and being positive is difficult; you are only human, and you will have days that test your positivity. In this instance, it is not a failure to explain to your staff that you are having a tough day. The best part of being a team is that you support one another, a team is not a top-down approach and there will be days where your team will help to improve your mood.

Try and smile even in the face of adversity; however, do make sure it is genuine. If you are not happy and cannot smile, remember it is okay to not be okay. Take a break and try and process what is causing you to feel this way. Reach out to another team member or to your senior to go through the problem and see if there is a solution. Being deliberately positive increases the mood in both you and your team. Smile to yourself now and notice how it increases your mood. Smiling makes you feel happier; feeling happier makes you smile!

Be aware that your facial expressions and body language affect the way the people around you feel and the way they work, this ultimately affects the standard of patient care. A positive attitude produces a good working atmosphere. It not only increases morale, but it also leads to increased performance and job satisfaction. Search for opportunities to invest in each person who works for you. See each inter-action with a member of your team as an opportunity to increase their positivity.

11.3.1 Be Optimistic

Being optimistic is not always an easy thing to be in a highly pressurised job, but it is important to try. This does not mean you have to think everything is wonderful, when you are actually struggling. What it does mean is that even in the hardest situations, you try and see the positives. For example, your ward is full and you are a member of staff short, but every person within the team has pulled together and has worked fantastically as a team. Some people would only see that the ward was full, and you were short staffed. What a good leader does is see how well the team coped in a difficult situation and came together to deliver the best care to patients. Take that opportunity to share this with your team. Explain that, even though it has been a hard shift, the dedication and hard work of the team made it the best of a bad situation and thank them.

11.3.2 Focus on the Solution, Not the Problem

Present solutions. There is usually something positive in any situation; you just need to draw it out. If you are greeted with a statement such as 'We are three staff down today and there are no agency available; how on earth are we going to cope?' do not let your facial expression fall with a reply like 'Oh no, I don't believe it'. Keep smiling, be positive and say something like 'Right, we'll have to make a list together of the tasks that we will leave undone, so that the patients are safe'.

Associate yourself with people who make you feel good. If your man-ager is one of those people whose glass is always half empty, listen and learn. Experiences with managers like this help you learn. Watch the effect that they are having, you will see firsthand how negativity breeds negativity. Strive to ensure you do not emulate such habits. You often learn how to be a good leader, from the mistakes of bad ones.

Luckily, the attributes of great leaders can be developed by anyone who is passionate and committed in their work. Start today by being cheerful, smiling and optimistic if you can, no matter what the situation you are in.

11.4 SPEAK CLEARLY

Your speaking style conveys more about you than maybe you would wish. People determine your intelligence, education, even your leadership ability by the words you use and by how you say them. The whole reason for speaking is to impart information clearly and effectively. If you tend to speak too softly or mumble, it could result in

- others not being able to hear or understand you;
- being misheard or misunderstood;
- giving the impression that you lack confidence;
- giving the impression that you do not really have anything interesting to say and so are insignificant.

If you stand upright with confidence, make eye contact and speak clearly, people will assume that you are knowledgeable and have something specific to say which is relevant to them. They will remember you. This skill does not always easily come to everyone, and if you relate to the statements above, it does not mean that you cannot be a good leader. Many trusts now run leadership courses, to help develop good leaders into great ones. Utilise these workshops, to help develop your skills.

11.4.1 Focus on Your Pronunciation

The nature of your role means you have to be able to think fast and make quick decisions throughout your shift. For some health workers, this comes out in their speech. It is a natural tendency to talk quickly when pressured or stressed. Speaking too quickly means that people cannot keep up with you, and there is a tendency to 'fall over' your words. The result is that not all of your message will get through. Some find it happens more often towards the end of the shift. Focusing on your pronunciation is a good way of slowing down your speech. People will be more attentive and more likely to understand what you are saying without having to ask you to repeat.

Concentrate on how you pronounce your words. Some people get into the habit of dropping the 'g's and 't's from the end of their words. This results in words being slurred together and can make you come across as uneducated. Say the following sentences out loud as if you were talking to one of your colleagues at work:

- 'Are you going to start the ward round in a minute?'
- 'Do you want to start taking your breaks now?'
- 'I'll sort out the discharge arrangements if you just take this phone call?'

Did you articulate each syllable and pronounce all the 'g's and 't's? Be aware that not doing so can inhibit you getting your message across clearly.

Filler phrases such as 'you know', 'actually' or lots of 'um's and 'er's also distract people from listening to what you are saying. People will notice these repetitive phrases more than they notice what you are saying.

11.4.2 Your Telephone Manner

The way you answer the telephone speaks volumes about you. Saying something like 'Ward 10?' is really not sufficient. 'Ward 10, Ward Manager speaking' is an improvement, but 'Ward 10, Ward Manager (your name) speaking. How may I help you?' is more warm and welcoming. It also makes you come across as confident and professional.

Body language is extremely important. The way you stand and the way you speak affect your total image. If you are constantly fidgeting or looking anywhere but at the person you are speaking to, you will appear ill at ease. This affects your telephone manner too. If you are slouched across the desk talking to someone over the phone, you will come across as less controlled than if you sit upright.

11.4.3 Stop Apologising

Be wary about apologising before you speak, and if you do tend to do this, try and break the habit unless you have genuinely done something to be sorry about. It can come across as if you are apologising for your presence and people are quick to pick up on that. Take the following examples:

- 'Sorry to bother you, would you mind taking one of our patients to theatre?'
- 'Sorry. I can see you are busy but Dr Smith has come to see Mrs Jones'.

If you find yourself using phrases such as those outlined above, try using the following alternative approaches:

- 'We have a patient ready for theatre. Is anyone available?'
- 'Excuse me interrupting you. Dr Smith is here to see Mrs Jones'.

These things may seem minor, but the way you convey yourself is so important if you want to be taken seriously.

And one last tip: in any professional context, swearing is not appropriate. When used *very* sparingly, it can have a powerful effect and make people take notice, but when used regularly, it will lower people's opinion of you and sets a bad example.

11.5 BE RELAXED AND IN CONTROL

If you are smart, articulate, always smiling and positive in your outlook, you will come across as warm, friendly and confident. In other words, you are creating the impression that you are in control; your work does not control you. Walk upright (no rounded shoulders) and greet people with a good strong handshake. It is an attractive quality; people are drawn to attractiveness.

11.5.1 Keep Yourself Cool

Never lose your temper. Loss of temper means loss of control. By all means, say how you feel but ensure you remain cool, calm and collected as you do so. There is nothing wrong with saying, 'I know you have a job to do, but I find your attitude quite unprofessional' and walking away if necessary. Do not get into a heated argument. It is unbecoming of a senior manager and will be talked about for years to come by the other party and any onlookers.

11.5.2 Manage Conflict With Confidence

It helps in times of conflict if you can identify whether you and the other party are adopting a parent, child or adult state. Eric Berne (a psychoanalyst who wrote the best-selling book called *Games People Play*) puts forward the theory that people tend to take on the persona of a parent, adult or child depending on what situation they are in (Berne, 1968). In times of conflict, try and decipher what role you are playing:

> *Parent state*: Are you nurturing the other person by trying to give advice or protect them by not giving enough responsibility? Are you being critical perhaps by telling them off for breaking the rules?
>
> *Child state*: Are you feeling insecure and expecting to be told what to do? Are you trying to rebel against 'the rules'?
>
> *Adult state*: Are you being sensible, calm and logical? Are you able to keep your emotions from interfering with the situation?

According to Berne, there is no 'best' or 'worst' state. Each can be helpful if used in the right situation. Being in 'adult mode', all the time can make for a very boring person. However, having an awareness of what state you and the other person are in can help you manage relationships more effectively.

Situations of conflict can be resolved by concentrating on bringing both parties into 'adult state'. If, for example, you have some members of your team who decide that they can behave how they like with complete disregard about the effects they have on others, you may be tempted to take on the role of the controlling parent. This can exacerbate the situation, whereas if you take on the adult role, which tends to be more unemotional and detached, it could help diffuse the situation and help produce a matching adult state in others.

11.5.3 Use of Empathy

Use of empathy is often a good way of resolving the situation if someone is being difficult. Being empathic means showing that you understand the other person's point of view by using phrases such as 'I understand what you are saying; I get frustrated with the system too sometimes'. Self-disclosure also helps. Tell them how their behaviour makes you feel, such as 'Your tone is making me feel uncomfortable'.

When you are in a situation of conflict, try and match the other person's parent or child state by empathising with them, then move them into more of an adult state by suggesting a joint solution. Using 'we' rather than 'you' or 'I' also helps in diffusing heated situations. This is illustrated in the following example:

> *Manager*: 'I'm not happy about the way you run the ward. You should not allow staff to be drinking coffee at the main reception desk'. *(Angry critical parent mode.)*

Sister: 'I can understand why you think like that. I feel the same myself at times'. *(Use of empathy and self-disclosure.)* 'The problem is when we are short staffed; the staff are unable to leave the ward for their breaks. Perhaps we could come up with an alternative solution?' *(Sensible adult mode, suggesting joint solution.)*

Whatever you do, always keep yourself cool. Working in healthcare, we are all subject to chronic staff shortages, bed pressures, poor resources and relentless performance targets. No wonder, working relationships are constantly put under strain. Some would say that conflict is inevitable, but if you keep yourself cool, it does not have to be.

Further tips that may help in times of adversity include the following:

1. Always manage difficult people face-to-face. Leaving voice mail, email, fax, notes, etc. will only serve to increase their animosity.
2. Control your own emotions; do not get angry and shout back. If you feel threatened or intimidated, say that you will leave and come back later when things have calmed down. Put some time and distance between the two of you. Never walk out in a huff.
3. Notice those in your team who are not being difficult, those who work hard and without complaint. Reward them. Just a simple thank you may be all that is needed. Do not allow the difficult ones to claim most of your attention.

11.6 MAKE YOUR WRITING DISTINGUISHABLE

How you write is very important, it is important that your writing is legible and free of acronyms where possible. This ensures that any documentation is accessible to anyone reading them.

11.6.1 Handwriting

Take the time to ensure that everything you write is

- neat and legible;
- consistent.

Make sure that your staff notice your handwriting, when they recognise it, they will notice the content. Your aim is for them to see your high standards of documentation.

In law, the clinical record portrays the standard of care. You should demonstrate a high standard of care at all times. Remember that patients' records are also reviewed by an array of health professionals – anaesthetists, surgeons, physiotherapists, complaints managers and even solicitors. They will all judge the standard of care based on the standard of your records. Ensure that as well as signing your writing, you write clearly your name and designation. The use of a stamp can help to ensure your name and designation is clear.

11.6.2 Care Plans and Evaluations

Unfortunately, the task of writing care plans and evaluations is still often relegated to the end of the shift. This is a time when people are tired and rushing to get everything done so that they can get home. It is not the best time to write such an important document. Demonstrate to your staff that they can make entries throughout the shift. Each time you complete an episode of care or if there is a change in the patient's condition, write an entry in the evaluation section (in your distinguishable handwriting). Obviously, it is not possible for you to do this each and every time, but try and get into the habit of writing your evaluations and any care plan updates throughout the shift rather than saving them all until the end. This is also recommended in principle 3 of the Record Keeping Guidance (Nursing and Midwifery Council, 2015). Make a particular point of doing this when you have a member of staff or student to shadow you for a shift.

11.6.3 E-mails

Emails are another area where it is wise to think how you would like others to email you. People will also judge your intellect through the way you write your emails. As a general rule:

- Go through your emails each day. Answer them as soon as you have time to dedicate to a response. If there is a delay, apologise.
- Always make the best use of the subject heading such as 'Re: Impending staffing shortage across medical unit next week' or 'Benchmarking meeting on Monday cancelled'. Subject headings like these mean your emails are more likely to be opened and noted.
- Make your emails easier to read by writing the most important information in the first paragraph and the background/supporting information in the rest of the email.
- Never use your work email account for private or personal emails. All your emails should come as no surprise if another member of your team gains access to them so treat emails, as if they are a postcard, anyone can read rather than a sealed letter. It is good development for a deputy or someone who is shadowing you for the day to go through your emails with you. It helps them to gain a good insight into your role and responsibilities.
- If the subject of your email is confidential, the majority of NHS-based emails are encrypted. If in any doubt, you can add an extra encryption code. If you are unsure as to how to do this, speak with your IT department.
- Do not send blind copies (bcc) casually. They imply that you are going behind someone's back.
- Do not ask for a receipt unless absolutely necessary. It implies that you do not trust the recipient to read or respond promptly to your emails.

- Use the urgent icon sparingly. If not, really urgent emails you send in the future may get overlooked.
- Do not use CAPITAL LETTERS. In email language, this is construed as SHOUTING!
- Always use a positive tone and be aware that the tone of emails can be misconstrued.
- Never leave your computer unattended, if you are to walk away, ensure you put a lock screen on. This is important for information governance.

Everything you write, whether by hand or computer, speaks volumes about you. Make sure you are conveying the right image and encourage others to have the same high standards.

11.7 BE AWARE OF HOW OTHERS SEE YOU

To be a good role model, you have to know yourself. Hopefully you know your strengths and weaknesses from your own point of view, but are you sure that others see you in the same light as you see yourself? How realistic is your image of yourself?

You may, for example, see one of your strengths as being assertive and getting things done, but others may regard you as aggressive and loud and as a result may shy away from you. You may feel that you are weak at organising your team, whereas your team may see it as a strength that you allow your team to organise their own work and make their own decisions.

There are now many different psychometric tests, the majority that are free to take, that you can take to give you a better understanding of your own personal characteristics. See also Chapter 12 for further information on DISC (Dominant, Influencer, Conscientious, Cautious) behavioural profiling.

11.7.1 Ask People to Point Out Your Key Strengths and Weaknesses

A simple way to find out what others think of you is to ask. Some recommend that you ask each of your peers, members of your team and your line manager to write down what they think your three key strengths are and identify one area that could be improved. This can be quite a humbling exercise, and some would have difficulty asking their colleagues what they think about them.

11.8 SET AN EXAMPLE WITH YOUR CHOICE OF LANGUAGE

Do not let negative people set the tone. There is always at least one person in a team who will consistently use language such as the following:

'We can't do that'.
'They'll never allow us to do that'.

'We've tried it all before, it won't work'.
'We've got enough to do'.
'We haven't got enough staff'.
'They don't know what it's like for us'.
'There's nothing we can do'.

These people have the attitude that someone else is always in control. They are not choosing what they do; other people rule their lives. They have a tendency to absolve responsibility for any choices they make.

Think about the language you use:

'I have to go to the sisters' meeting this afternoon'.
'We have to do it this way because …'
'I've tried but it makes no difference'.
'If only we could recruit one more member of staff'.

Using language like this will give the impression you are not in control. Not only that, others may adopt this negative tone. Think carefully about the language you use, make sure others see you as someone who is in control of the situation. Managers will often use negative phrases to cover up their guilt at leaving staff extra work in their absence. Instead, just explain why you have chosen to go to the meeting: 'I shall be leaving you this afternoon for a couple of hours to attend a meeting about the future changes within the directorate'. This is just as acceptable but shows that you are in charge of what you are doing.

Try to use positive language such as the following:

'What is the alternative?'
'I will …'
'I choose to …'
'I prefer to …'
'I shall …'
'OK, so that didn't work, what shall we try instead?'
'I have decided to …'
'I am going to …'

Making subtle changes in your way of thinking and you change your way of seeing things and the way others see you.

11.9 NEVER MOAN OR GOSSIP ABOUT OTHERS

Try and keep negative opinions to yourself. Do not get pulled into a situation where a group of staff sit around talking about individuals who are not present to defend themselves. Retrain yourself to look for the good in each person and in each situation. Change the conversation around by pointing out the positive things about the individual or change the subject completely. If you gossip, your staff will gossip. As their role model, think about what behaviour you are portraying to them.

Moaning and gossiping about others is contagious and achieves nothing. Once one person starts, others join in and it creates an overall negative atmosphere. Your job is to try and maintain a continual positive atmosphere. In addition to this, if you do speak negatively about others, your staff may well think, 'If my manager says this about others, what is said about me when my back is turned?'

People are wary when in the company of gossips and will not talk freely. As a manager, you need to be seen as someone that people can be open and honest with. Being heard gossiping will only hinder you. Socialising with your staff is perfectly acceptable and should be encouraged, but remember that you are still their manager and that how you would be in work is still applicable to outside of work.

11.9.1 Moaning About Work

If you find yourself moaning about work, make yourself think of a solution to the issue instead. Sometimes there may not be a solution to the issue, if this is the case, express your frustration to your manager, and move forward. If there is a solution, put your efforts into solving the issue instead of wasting your valuable time moaning about it. People tend to moan or procrastinate when faced with

- a large workload;
- unrealistic time commitments;
- too many interruptions;
- work requiring skills they do not have.

If this is happening to your team regularly, perhaps you need to take a step back and look at what you and your team can do to control your workload rather than allowing it to control you (see Chapter 2).

11.9.2 Change the Moaning Culture

If you are one of those people whose glass is more half empty than half full, try and make a conscious effort to look on the bright side. People are much more likely to warm to you if you are talking positively rather than negatively. Get into the habit of it and you will not only give yourself a lift, but others too.

Make the staff room a nice place to be in by adding things that lift people's spirits. Put photos on the wall from ward nights out. Ensure there are nice mugs for tea rather than drab paper cups. Make sure there is always a plentiful supply of coffee, tea, sugar and milk. Perhaps even get the staff to add an extra £1 to the kitty, and when things are particularly challenging, buy some cream cakes for the team. These may seem small gestures but together they will help to prevent a climate of moaning and gossiping and general dissatisfaction.

11.10 DO NOT STAGNATE

Demonstrate a personal commitment to improving yourself and others by showing that you are continually willing to learn and develop professionally. Methods you can use to role model that commitment are through

- sharing your learning and experiences;
- involvement in the wider organisation;
- involvement in wider professional issues;
- having others shadow you.

11.10.1 Sharing Your Learning and Experiences

If you personally attend any courses, teaching sessions or conferences, make a point of sharing what you have learned with the rest of your team. If you have a patient with a condition rarely seen by the team, find out about it and share the knowledge with your team. Do not just encourage others to do this. Show them the way and how it should be done. Your staff will be more willing to share what they have learned with the team if they observe you doing it all the time.

Always practice what you preach. Most nurses remember being told to share their learning as a student or junior staff nurse. It can cause a lot of unnecessary anxiety for them if they are the only ones required to do this. If you and your senior staff put on sessions regularly where you share your learning, it will become common practice and junior staff will be more willing to take part.

11.10.2 Involvement in the Wider Organisation

Becoming involved in hospital committees not only widens your networks, but it can also help your staff to broaden their horizons too. Take one of them along with you to the meetings every now and then to introduce them to the higher 'workings' of the organisation. Show them just how important your meetings are and how they influence clinical practice.

Demonstrating to your staff how influential you are at a higher level gives them an insight as to how influential they can be in their future careers. Give them firsthand knowledge of any decisions made and how and why they will affect future practice. Seeing you have wider influence will increase their respect in your skills and abilities too.

11.10.3 Involvement in Wider Professional Issues

Make sure you are a member or are involved in the professional association linked with your role. If you do not have a specialist association, try other professional bodies. The Royal College of Nursing (RCN) holds various management and leadership forums with which you could become involved. Another option is to join a community group to help develop the links with the community teams.

Do not become involved in any more than two groups at the very most. It would not be appropriate to allow outside commitments to interfere with your day-to-day managerial responsibilities.

11.10.4 Having Others Shadow You

Encourage members of your staff (registered, unregistered and students) to shadow you regularly if you can. Having someone to shadow you will help to keep you up-to-date. They will ask questions and make you think about the way you work. Having to explain why you make decisions stimulates you to think again about why you do things. It is hard work and can be quite challenging but is an enormous benefit to your learning. You can also learn new ideas from those that shadow you. They will be fresh with ideas from other wards where they have worked or with new techniques and knowledge from various courses or study they have undertaken.

Never think you know everything. No matter how long you have been in your job or specialty, there is always more to learn. It is advisable to adopt this attitude at all times. If you still have lots to learn, then your staff will too. If you allow yourself to stagnate, your staff will follow suit.

11.10.4.1 Action Points

- Check your uniform policy and make sure you strictly adhere to it as an example to others.
- Make a point of warmly greeting all visitors to your ward and focus the conversation on them.
- Start smiling more and focusing on the positive aspects in all situations.
- Speak slowly, clearly and focus on pronouncing your 'g's and 't's, particularly if you have a tendency to talk quickly.
- In times of conflict, try and identify what state you and the other person are in – parent, child or adult. Use empathy and self-disclosure to bring both into an adult state.
- Think of ways you can get feedback from your team (in a nonthreatening manner) to identify areas you can improve upon.
- Stop yourself each time you say 'I can't' or 'I have to' and change it to 'I will' or 'I choose to'.
- If you have a tendency to gossip or moan about things at work, think about why you do this and what you can do to stop this habit.
- Consider ways in which you can demonstrate to others that you are continually learning by sharing your experiences.

REFERENCES

Berne, E., 1968. Games People Play. Penguin, London.
Nursing and Midwifery Council, 2015. Record Keeping: Guidance for Nurses and Midwives. NMC, London.

Chapter 12

Manage Your Manager

A very important, but much neglected, part of being a good manager is building up a good working relationship with your own manager. This may not seem your foremost concern because you are focussing so much on building your own team. But if you make time for your manager, you will ensure that you

- are more likely to be involved in making important decisions that affect your team;
- have greater access to appropriate help to achieve your team's goals;
- gain respect and are taken seriously;
- learn from your manager's experiences (including mistakes);
- keep well informed;
- have greater freedom and authority to act.

If you do not put time and effort into building up a good working relationship with your manager, you can become low on their priority list.

Having a poor relationship with your manager does you no favours at all. It will hinder your progress. It does not matter whether you like them or not; they have knowledge, experience and information that you do not. You should find the right ways of working with them to help achieve yours and their goals.

12.1 CLARIFY EXPECTATIONS

In a manner of speaking, having a line manager means you are a follower and followers need three clarities:

Clarity of purpose: This is your 'why', your purpose for doing what you do. It is more than your technical purpose of leading your unit; it relates to your values, your aspirations and your vision for your unit.

Clarity of plan: This is your 'how' and your 'what'. It is the technical part of how you deliver your goals with your team and for the organisation.

Clarity of responsibility: This is your 'who' and articulates the difference of roles, who does what and is for responsible for which elements of the role. Establishing this with both your manager and your own team at all levels enables everyone to feel safer in the knowledge that they know what is expected as problems can arise if there is a lack of clarity between you about your tasks and responsibilities.

12.1.1 Understanding Different Personality Types

It is common at senior leader level to undertake psychometric testing, such as Myers Briggs Type Indicator (MBTI), as part of an interview process, it is important to appreciate that not everyone sees the world the same way that you do. DISC is a behaviour assessment tool based on the DISC theory of psychologist William Moulton Marston, which centres on four different personality traits, which are currently Dominance (D), Influence (I), Steadiness (S), and Conscientiousness (C). The elements are as follows:

Dominance:

> Driven
> Results oriented
> Firm
> Strong-willed
> Forceful

Influencer

> Outgoing
> Enthusiastic
> Optimistic
> High-spirited
> Lively

Steady

> Even-tempered
> Accommodating
> Patient
> Humble
> Tactful

Conscientious

> Analytical
> Reserved
> Precise
> Private
> Systematic

Task-oriented people, that is, those who are predominantly Dominant and/or Conscientious tend to focus on logic, data, results and projects. People-oriented people, that is, those who are predominantly Influencer and/or Steady tend to focus on experiences, feelings, relationships and interactions with other people. DISC provides a common language people can use to better understand themselves and others, and it is important to stress that we are not one-dimensional but a blend of all four types with a preference for one or two elements in particular.

There are no 'good' or 'bad' personality types, only strengths and weaknesses, and personality is never an excuse for poor behaviour.

12.1.2　Be Clear About What You Expect From Your Manager

You do not have to become a great friend with your manager, but it is important to understand their role and the demands placed on them. If you know what the organisation expects from your manager, then you will understand more readily why they work the way they do and why they make the decisions they do.

Your manager may have a different management style to you. They may be used to giving out orders and telling people what to do rather than involving the team in any decision-making. This may not sit well with you. If that is the case, then say so, but do not jump in with both feet. After all, their style may emanate from their own lack of confidence, so to 'attack' them may be counterproductive. Likewise, you may be construed as being secretive if your own style is like that identified above. Notwithstanding this, be clear about both your expectations of each other to be involved, not just informed.

Ask your manager for regular feedback, both positive and negative, so that you can continuously improve in your work, rather than wait for your annual appraisal to find out how you are progressing.

Make sure you get your appraisal each year. Do not wait for your manager to initiate the process. Write down what you want to discuss:

1. Your own self-assessment on how you think you are doing.
2. The objectives you feel are the priorities for your ward.
3. Your personal development needs to achieve those objectives.

You need to understand what your manager's own objectives are too. A good manager will ensure that your objectives reflect their own. In that way, you will know that you are both heading in the same direction. It would be detrimental if your objectives were totally different from those of your manager. That would only serve to create tension in your working relationship, not to mention the effect on practice.

Remember that your manager is only human. Sometimes, people are labelled as 'poor' managers because they do not conform to our expectations. Your manager may have become out of touch clinically, for example, but may still be particularly good at helping you to write complaint letters or getting more resources for your ward. Make sure you get the most from what they do well and try not to focus on any weaknesses.

12.1.3　Be Clear About What Your Manager Expects From You

Your manager will probably have managed a ward or department before their promotion. Problems sometimes occur when they expect you to manage your ward in the same way that they did. One of the ways you can manage that is to keep your manager fully informed about what you are doing. Show what you are doing well. Be clear about the skills you have and those you want to improve upon. Your manager usually needs to believe in your abilities before they will trust you.

If your manager does not communicate their expectations clearly, then it is your responsibility to ask what is expected. Your manager may not have good management or support from their own manager; this may affect their own ability to manage you. You need to appreciate their position and accept that they may need prompting to articulate their expectations. Make sure you have what your manager expects in terms of organisational objectives written down clearly during your appraisal. Always refer to these in anything that you do. If your manager comes to you with further projects, ask yourself whether it relates to your original objectives. If it does not, question your manager's expectations. Are they perhaps too high?

Try not to get into the habit of propping up a failing or struggling manager. Encourage them to get help and support from elsewhere. You cannot provide your manager with the same support that you give your team. It is not fair on you and you must let them know that.

12.2 WORK WITH, NOT AGAINST, YOUR MANAGER

Just because someone is your manager, it does not mean that they are perfect and know everything. Like you, they will also be learning from their experiences and mistakes. Do not focus on their weaknesses; nobody is perfect. Focus on their strengths; they would not be in the job if they did not do a great deal right.

12.2.1 Meet Regularly

Have regular meetings to review your objectives. Take the initiative and set up these meetings if your manager does not already do so. The constant changes in healthcare, including the ever-changing contracts and performance indicators, may result in a need for you to change your priorities. Make sure any changes to priorities are discussed and objectives changed and agreed accordingly. Without keeping a regular check on them, you could find you are going in a different direction to your manager.

12.2.2 Remain Loyal

If you do not like the way your manager works, do something about it. Tell your manager how you feel and suggest ways of changing their approach. Do not complain to others about their way of working. You must be seen to be working on the side of your manager at all times. Both their managers and employees alike can never trust disloyal people. A reputation for disloyalty can be hard to dispel.

12.2.3 Clarifying Role Boundaries Between You and Your Manager

If you feel your manager is interfering too much in clinical issues, you need to ask yourself why. Are you showing them what a good job you do or are you leaving it up to them to find out? Managers do not have time to constantly observe their employees. Take the initiative; keep them abreast of what you do well and any achievements regularly. They will appreciate more of what you do, rather than what you do not do.

Some managers struggle to let go of the clinical side, particularly if they have been promoted internally. Sometimes this means they do not have confidence in their more senior role and are taking refuge in what they do know. The key in this situation is to give consistent positive feedback on what they are doing well and then intersperse this with some feedback about how their additional involvement on the clinical side is affecting you and your team in a nonproductive way. Having a discussion around clarity of responsibility incorporates a boundaries conversation. It is important to respect and tap into the clinical expertise your manager may have and it should be welcomed; however, their role is not a clinical one in the way that yours is and their clinical knowledge will inevitably degrade over time so be kind too as if you moved from one clinical speciality to another, you would find yourself in the same position.

12.2.4 Assist in Decision-Making

Some managers find it difficult to decide what to do when confronted with a problem, particularly when clinical skills have become 'rusty'. The best thing you can do in this situation is to help them by outlining the possible solutions, making it clear to them which one you feel is the most suited at that time. You may need to follow this up with clear directions on the steps that need to be taken. Remember always to support them in any decision they make, including the 'fall-out' should it be the wrong decision. Nobody ever wants to hear the phrase 'I told you so' or 'It was the manager's decision, not mine'.

12.2.5 What if Your Manager Is Always Too Busy?

Being permanently busy does not mean that more work is getting done. It can sometimes mean the person is not in control of their workload. If your manager is busy and not in control, it will probably affect your work too. Meeting with your manager to confirm what you have defined as your workload (as outlined in Chapter 2) may help them to see that it would be a good idea for them to do the same exercise.

Every time your manager comes to you saying, 'We have to do this ... ' (e.g. another audit, a new procedure or a further reduction in staffing levels), ask yourself three questions:

1. 'Do we *have* to do this, or do we *choose* to do this?' (if you do not choose to do it, you are not in control), then:
2. 'If we choose not to do this, what will the intended or unintended consequences be?'
3. 'If we choose to do this, how much time and resources will it take, and which of our current tasks will we discontinue in order to make time for the new more important task?'

12.3 ACT, IF AN IMPORTANT DECISION HAS BEEN MADE WITHOUT YOUR CONSULTATION

If any important changes need to be made at work, everyone should be consulted. You should be given the chance to say what you think, and your manager should genuinely listen, consider and respond to your views.

Do not always blame others if you were left out from a decision-making process; you have to shoulder some of the responsibility. Ask yourself why you were not included. Do not get angry, do not procrastinate and do not bottle it up. Go and speak to your manager before you speak to anyone else. Remain calm and ask why you were not consulted. They may have simply forgotten and more often than not it is a simple human oversight not a conspiracy.

If you have views or alternative solutions, then let them know. If you feel there will be serious consequences that may not have been considered, make these very clear. Follow up your discussion with an email confirming what you discussed. You can address the email to any others involved in the decision-making process, so that they may also consider your views, but if you do, you should consider your wording very carefully. Avoid giving the impression that you are being disloyal to your manager. Ultimately you may not be able to change the decision made, but it helps if your views are made clear and considered.

12.3.1 Prevent It Happening Again

Treat this as a learning experience and take action to reduce the risk of it happening again. If you find that your manager genuinely forgot to include you or did not realise the importance of involving you, it may be a sign that you have not been making enough effort to communicate with them on a regular basis. Make sure you do so in future.

Do not just contact your manager when you have a problem or when they call a meeting. Make the effort to see your line manager regularly to update them on current issues. Keep them informed of everything you are doing. It is also important to keep them up to date with any projects or work that have been delegated to you.

Nurses are generally not good at promoting themselves, but if you do not promote your knowledge, expertise and how your team is doing, how else is your manager going to know? It is not sufficient to say that it is their job to find out. It is also your job to let them know and get yourself involved in activities, meetings and projects in which your knowledge and expertise are required.

12.3.2 Organisation-Wide Decisions

Financial and performance pressures and an unrelenting focus from national regulators, politicians and the media all compete for the limited time that senior NHS executives have (Anandaciva et al., 2018). You will need to translate the trust's plans into goals for your team and review progress in regular team meetings. Consider how you can share this information with the whole team to help members understand why it is important. Your meetings with your manager should include a discussion about the organisational objectives and how your team is supporting delivery (NHS Improvement, 2018a,b).

12.3.3 Is It Bullying?

If you feel you are doing everything you can to improve communications with your manager but feel that you are being deliberately left out of decision-making, this could be construed as bullying. It is advisable in this situation that you keep file notes. Record all incidents where you have not been consulted and note all actions you have taken to try to improve the situation.

Try and speak to your manager first. Tell them how their actions are making you feel. Discuss your concerns and agree on actions to be taken in the future. If your manager refuses to change or even to listen to you, seek further advice from a senior HR advisor. They will guide you through the process outlined in your local policy for bullying and harassment. They will also provide you with support and access to counselling if required.

12.4 ACT, IF A CHANGE IN ANOTHER DEPARTMENT HAS A KNOCK-ON EFFECT IN YOURS

Healthcare is continually changing to meet differing demands, with performance indicators and financial restrictions complicating the process. Decisions may have to be made quickly, and sometimes they are not properly thought through. Certain aspects can be overlooked, particularly the effects on neighbouring departments.

Mistakes happen, and a common example is disruption through building work. The facilities department may be doing building work nearby and you find the noise is intolerable for patients returning from, for instance, the operating theatre who need optimum rest to recover.

Shouting at a member of the facilities department over the telephone will probably have little effect and it is not even remotely professional. Gather your information or data first. Find out:

- Who else is affected?
- Are they suffering in silence too?
- What has anyone else tried to do about it?
- Who is the senior person in charge of the project?
- Was your line manager(s) involved or consulted?

It is sometimes the case that the manager was consulted and gave permission for the work to go ahead but genuinely forgot to inform everyone concerned or did not realise the impact of the decision on the wards. If this is the case, contacting the manager of the facilities department first is not appropriate. Your manager should be the first person to contact.

Do not just complain to your line manager and expect them to resolve the issue. State the problem and work together on possible solutions. Present your case together to the appropriate manager of the building works project, preferably face-to-face, and follow up your discussion and agreed actions with an email. Keep your line manager informed and involved at each stage in the process.

Remember to always keep records and copies of emails. Suggest solutions once you have all the facts, such as cancelling surgery, closing beds and transferring patients to other wards temporarily. Work with the facilities manager and your own line manager in finding suitable solutions. Do not focus on the fact that you were not consulted in the planning process.

12.4.1 Emergency Situations

In emergency situations, you have no choice. If you have to take a number of patients who require additional care and need to book extra agency staff, then so be it. But make it clear in such situations that you do not have the funds within your budget to deal with these extra demands. Work out afterwards, with the help of your finance advisor, roughly what the cost will be and inform your line manager. Make sure your discussion is documented and a copy sent to your line manager and whoever else is involved in making the decision including your Divisional Manager and Director of Nursing.

12.4.2 Safe Staffing

Safe staffing means having enough nurses with the right skills and knowledge, in the right place, at the right time. It is much more than about numbers; it includes the right skill mix including that of other disciplines, such as medicine and allied health, as well as patient acuity and case mix. As the ward leader, you will be responsible for assessing the factors that determine nursing staff requirements.

You need to understand your organisation's approach and learn how you can effectively demonstrate the needs of your ward. Factors you need to consider include the following:

- Use individual patients' nursing needs as the main factor for calculating the nursing staff requirements for a ward.
- Assess each patient's nursing needs holistically and take account of specific nursing requirements and disabilities, as well as other patient factors that may increase nursing staff requirements, such as:
  - difficulties with cognition or confusion (such as those associated with learning difficulties, mental health problems or dementia);
  - end-of-life care;
  - increased risk of clinical deterioration;
  - need for a nursing team member to be continuously present, referred to as enhanced care.
- Expected patient turnover in the ward during a 24-h period (including planned and unscheduled admissions, discharges and transfers).
- Ward layout and size (including the need to ensure the safety of patients who cannot be easily observed and the distance needed to travel to access resources within the ward) (NHS Improvement, 2018a; NICE, 2014).

It is important to be clear about the safe staffing roles and responsibilities for each level of nursing leadership in your organisation:

Ward manager – remains accountable for providing safe staffing levels to meet patient needs and service demands and should ensure the duty roster reflects the agreed workforce model.

Matron – responsible for ensuring each ward is safely staffed in their speciality. Where the ward manager identifies risks, the matron should seek to assist in any mitigation strategies to ensure all rosters are safe and meet patient needs and service demands, escalating any safety issues to their heads of nursing.

Heads of nursing – responsible for ensuring all wards in their division are safely staffed and all risks have been minimised. It is the head of nursing's responsibility to ensure the deputy chief nurse/chief nurse is informed.

Chief nurse – executive director responsible for overall safe staffing on the wards and departments across the trust. It is their responsibility to report to the board on the safe staffing position (NHS Improvement, 2018b).

12.4.3 Project Work

If you are asked to take on a piece of work on behalf of the directorate or the organisation, such as an audit, clarify how much time and resources it will take (remember that staff time is a resource). If you are required to undertake the work personally, identify and agree with your manager which aspect of your existing workload you will prioritise, to make time to do this extra work. Even a piece of work such as investigating a complaint or incident for another area could take a few days or weeks.

If members of your team are required to do extra work such as new link nurse roles or attending organisation-wide working groups, calculate how many hours' work will be required and work out how much that will cost you in terms of clinical cover.

If a member of staff needs to take on a new link nurse role, for example, work out how much time they will need to fulfil the role. It may need the link nurse to:

- attend a 2-h meeting each month;
- take follow-up actions from each meeting;
- keep the ward team informed and up-to-date regularly;
- deliver teaching sessions.

The above tasks may require the equivalent of 1–2 days' worth of additional work per month. How much will this cost in terms of agency cover? Even if you find the link nurse stays on for a short time after each shift to fulfil the duties required and accrues time owed, the time they eventually take will come out of your budget. It costs money to cover a shift or half a shift when the nurse takes her time back. There is usually no allowance within your funded establishment to cover 'time owed' unless this is agreed with your line manager and the finance department (see Chapter 6).

12.4.4 When You Are 'Micromanaged'

Working with a manager who micromanages you, that is, checks up on everything and feels the need to obsessively control every minute detail can be stressful. Managers who micromanage can also rob their team of the opportunity to grow and develop their own skills and can lead to paralysis of decision-making in your own work environment.

Micromanagement rarely has to do with your performance and more often relates to their own internal anxiety and need to control situations. It is worth remembering that there are two ends of the micromanagement spectrum; those with very high standards (think Apple's Steve Jobs) and they pay great attention to details. You may learn a great deal from them. The other end is those who are not too subtly indicating they need to be in total charge of everything and they are much more difficult to handle.

Here are a number of principles to remember
Do's:

- Do everything you can to gain the micromanager's trust.
- Know what motivates and worries your boss and try to assuage his/her concerns.
- Provide regular and detailed updates so your boss is apprised of your progress

Don'ts:

- Label anyone who exercises a degree of control as a micromanager.
- Defy the micromanager-that often triggers the behaviour you are trying to avoid.
- Try to tell a boss that he/she is overly controlling unless you know he/she may be open to hearing it.

12.4.5 Keep in Constant Contact and Give Feedback

Contact your manager regularly, at least once a week, and give them a general update. This will ensure they are aware of the good practice on your ward and will remember to keep you involved in wider issues. It is a good idea to give your line manager regular feedback just as you do with your team. You want to be able to encourage all the positive aspects of their behaviour and make them aware of aspects which have a negative effect. If your manager comes to see you regularly each week and you appreciate that, say so. If your manager has a tendency to interfere unnecessarily with the work of your team, your frustration may not be understood unless you say so. In this case, the manager may think they are help-ing you and could have no idea unless you maintain an open and honest dialogue.

Similarly, try to encourage some feedback from your manager so that you have some idea how you are progressing. Some managers may not give feed-back unless asked.

12.5 WRITE CLEAR AND TIMELY REPORTS

Getting reports finished on time and done properly will help enormously in building a good relationship with your manager. Try not to put all report-writing tasks to the bottom of your in-tray. Start the process immediately as it prevents you spending time worrying about when you are going to get the time to do it. Developing a basic outline to start with should help you to be clearer in your mind about what information is required and you may even be able to delegate parts of the report where appropriate.

When asked by your line manager to write a report, confirm the objective of the report and who the reader(s) will be before you start work on it. Taking time to check this at the beginning can save you hours of wasted effort later on. It should help you to decide what information to include or leave out, and hope-fully prevent your manager saying after all your hard work, 'This is not what I asked for'.

12.5.1 Stage 1: Write a Basic Outline

Write a basic outline before you start researching or investigating the informa-tion that you will need. It will help direct your investigation. All reports should be based on the following headings, which can be individually adapted at a later stage:

1. Executive summary (and recommendations if any).
2. Introduction (based on the objective).
3. Background (include the method of investigation/research).
4. Results (and any implementation).
5. Conclusion.

Start any report with these five basic headings to guide you. It prevents you from sitting down and staring at a piece of blank paper wondering where to begin.

12.5.2 Stage 2: The Introduction

The introduction is one of the most important sections of a report. The reader can form an opinion about the rest of the report based on the clarity and quality of the introduction. It is a good idea to use the objective you have agreed with your manager to form the basis of the introduction to your report.

12.5.3 Stage 3: Background Description

Describe the background to the report, that is, make the context clear. Keep it in note form in the initial stages to stop you becoming too focussed on this section. If your report is about how you have done something to come up with a solution, use this section to describe the process you used. It is often better to complete this section once you have finished the rest of the report.

12.5.4 Stage 4: Results/Implementation

This is the main part of the report. A good idea to get started is to list everything you want to include in the report, and then group points into key headings. You could write down each item on a 'post-it' note, and then sort the 'post-it' notes into general themes or key headings. Once you have done this, you can concentrate on researching or finding the information to put in under each heading and delegating some parts to your team or others if appropriate.

12.5.5 Stage 5: Conclusion and Recommendations

Use this section to conclude the main findings or recommendations.

12.5.6 Stage 6: Executive Summary

It is easier to write this after writing the report, although it needs to be inserted at the beginning. It should be a brief summary, ideally on one page of the report with any recommendations. This should enable the reader to get an overview of what is in the report without having to read it through.

12.5.6.1 Further Tips

When you come to the writing part, there are a few rules to remember:

1. Write in the first person, 'I'; not 'one' or 'the author'.
2. Do not use jargon such as 'obs' or 'resps'.
3. Use active, not passive, phrases (e.g. 'we decided' rather than 'it was decided').
4. Avoid exclamation marks.
5. Try to avoid using superfluous phrases such as 'at this moment in time' instead of 'now', or 'in respect of' instead of 'about', 'use' instead of 'utilise'.
6. Paragraphs should be wider than they are long.
7. Explain all abbreviations, keeping in mind that some people who read the report will not be healthcare professionals.
8. Ensure the report has page numbers.

As a general rule, any reports should be short and succinct and include more facts than descriptions. Few managers will read long reports from cover to cover. Most will read the introduction, key headings, conclusion and recommendations, so concentrate on those aspects.

Always give reports in on time. Managers are usually impressed by people who deliver work early or on time.

12.6 KNOW HOW TO CONDUCT A GOOD INVESTIGATION

You may be asked by your line manager to undertake a full investigation into matters involving issues such as

- conduct concerns;
- capability concerns;
- grievances;
- complaints;
- allegation of bullying and harassment;
- whistleblowing (speak-up) concerns

Usually you would not undertake a formal investigation into staff behaviour on your own ward. It is good practice to appoint investigators who are not involved in the incident or line-manage the area in which the involved member(s) of staff work. (Remember that complaint and incident investigations are not formal and therefore require a different informal investigation, which is usually carried out by you and your team in your own area.)

Before commencing any formal investigation, confirm the following with your manager:

1. Exactly what is to be investigated and under which policy.
2. The time frame for completion. You will need to negotiate dedicated time in which to carry out the investigation. Do not attempt to do this in your own time, or in quiet times during your shift. You may require cover for your time out.
3. Who you can go to for support. You should have access to an experienced HR advisor throughout the process.

12.7 GUIDING PRINCIPLES OF INVESTIGATIONS

Investigations should

- be impartial, objective and be underpinned by openness and transparency;
- be carried out promptly;
- incorporate relevant documentary evidence;
- incorporate witness and interview statements from all relevant parties;
- seek to establish and set out the facts;
- highlight any conflicts in evidence collated;
- draw logical conclusions on conflicting evidence on the standard of 'balance of probability';
- result in a report that draws logical conclusion based on the evidence collated.

12.7.1 Make a Provisional Plan of Action

Agree on a plan of action with your manager. This plan may change as new information comes to light, but you should start off with a plan, so you can estimate the time it will take.

Your first step in your plan is usually to arrange the interview dates. It takes considerable time to arrange venues, dates and times. Do not carry out the interviews until you have reviewed all the necessary documentary evidence, but try and do them as quickly as possible after the event to

- ensure the event(s) is still fresh in everyone's mind;
- stop rumours and gossip;
- reduce unnecessary anxiety for all those involved;
- reduce unnecessary waste of resources if anyone has been suspended.

When you arrange the interviews, you must ensure that each person is informed of their right to have a trade union representative or work colleague to accompany them. It is up to them to arrange this. You should also let them know of any support that your organisation offers such as trained counsellors for victims of alleged bullying. You should ensure that the alleged wrongdoer is informed in writing of the investigation and the subject of said investigation as soon as possible. It is an expectation under the NMC Code (2015) that nurses will cooperate with any internal and external investigations. It would be unfair for the witnesses or anyone else to hear of the investigation before them. You should also keep the ward/department manager informed as well as your own line manager.

12.7.2 Review All the Documentary Evidence

It is advisable to make photocopies of any documentary evidence to prevent tampering of records. Keep a record of all documents reviewed as part of the process. Relevant documents may include the following:

- rosters
- ward induction/development programmes
- patients' medical or nursing records
- local policies/guidelines
- any relevant professional or national guidelines

Remember to follow the confidentiality guidelines if any patient information is required for the investigation (see Chapter 7).

12.7.3 Interviews

Interviews usually start with the person who raised the issue. This is to establish the nature of the complaint or allegation and any further information that may be relevant. You will also need to interview the alleged wrongdoer(s) to give them the chance to put across their version of events. Any witnesses will need to be interviewed as well as the line manager. If you are investigating a matter of which you have no knowledge or experience, you may also need to interview other professionals for their expert advice. Witnesses are usually entitled to time off in lieu or payment if interviewed outside of normal working hours. Check your organisational policy and inform their line managers of the time required if this is the case.

Before you start an interview, you should prepare your questions to ensure you cover all the required areas. At the beginning of the interview, take time to do the following:

1. Make the person feel comfortable with appropriate refreshments and seating.
2. Reiterate their right to be accompanied by a trade union representative or work colleague.
   Explain that this is not disciplinary action and that your role is only to establish the facts. That noted, remind them that although formal sanctions such as a verbal or written warning cannot be imposed at an investigatory meeting, the investigation can trigger the disciplinary process and possibly lead to disciplinary action being taken.

3. Explain that they should not discuss the case with anyone else who is involved.

Keep a record of all the interviews. Give each person the opportunity to read through the notes of their interview and sign that they agree it is an accurate reflection of what was discussed; however, do not pressure them to sign notes at the meeting itself. They may prefer to provide their own statements. Make sure they are aware that any statements may be used as evidence in the event of a subsequent disciplinary hearing.

Advise people they may need to be recalled for further interviews and you may find you have to do this as further information comes to light. Remember that all information obtained should remain confidential so do not share information about anyone else's interview with subsequent interviewees. In practice, this can be quite difficult to achieve so be vigilant.

12.7.4 Prepare a Written Report

The following headings can be used as a general guide, but check your organisation's policy for local guidance on what is expected within your report:

- Executive summary (no more than 10 lines).
- Introduction – include terms of reference or objective.
- Description of the issue and/or allegations and an outline of the investigative process including timetable of interviews.
- Findings – list them clearly. You may wish to list them under headings of each complaint. Refer to witnesses either by their initials or as witness A, B or C, etc. throughout the report.
- Conclusions – is the complaint or allegation substantiated?
- Recommendations.
- Appendices.

The purpose of an investigation is to establish the facts. It does not equate to disciplinary action. It may or may not lead to a disciplinary hearing. If it does, the evidence provided in the investigative report will help inform the disciplinary panel.

12.8 ACTION POINTS

- If you have not already had one within the past year, make an appointment with your manager for an appraisal and ensure your objectives are congruent with theirs.
- Arrange regular meetings with your manager throughout the rest of the year to review your set objectives and to keep them informed of progress on your ward.

- If your manager leaves you out of decision-making or any changes, make a point of trying to improve your working relationship with them to reduce the risk of it happening again.
- If a change takes place that is detrimental to patient care, gather the facts and approach the appropriate people with the support of your manager.
- Try not to present any problems to your manager; present solutions or options for action each time.
- Give regular feedback to your manager, particularly with a job done well. Invite lots of feedback from your manager to ensure you are continually improving your own performance.
- Take on the delegation of an investigation as a challenge and opportune learning experience.
- Always start reports early and give them in early or on time.

REFERENCES

Anandaciva, S., Ward, D., Randhawa, M., Edge, R., 2018. Leadership in Today's NHS: Delivering the Impossible. King's Fund, London.

NHS Improvement, 2018a. The Ward Leaders Handbook. NHS Improvement, London.

NHS Improvement, 2018b. Developing Workforce Safeguards: Supporting Providers to Deliver High Quality Care through Safe and Effective Staffing. NHS Improvement, London.

National Institute for Health and Care Excellence (NICE), 2014. Safe Staffing for Nursing in Acute Adult Inpatient Wards in Hospitals. NICE, London.

Nursing and Midwifery Council, 2015. The Code: Professional Standards of Practice and Behaviour for Nurses and Midwives. NMC, London.

Chapter 13

Manage Difficult Situations

Managers, including you, have to deal with all sorts of different personalities ranging from the shy and passive to the explosive and aggressive types. Working in the healthcare environment can bring out the worst as well as the best in people as the pressure increases with more work and fewer resources. It is important to understand the emotional vulnerability that underlies many difficult situations. A key managerial skill is the ability to notice individual needs for recognition and self-esteem and to be confident in confronting challenging situations and people in a constructive and positive manner.

13.1 THE DIFFICULT MANAGER

People usually get promoted because they are good at their job, although it is not uncommon to be promoted after a period of acting up to cover someone who has left the organization, sickness/parental leave who then does not return. The challenge for clinicians being good at their job is that when promoted to become managers, they find it is a totally different job from that which they were doing before, and they do not necessarily have the skills in managing people or resources. (In some cases, people are promoted because they are poor clinicians or because they have been in the organisation for a very long time, but thankfully this is rarer nowadays.) Most managers thrive and with experience and support become even better over time. Unfortunately, there are a few who do not. Some will struggle in their role and may take out their frustrations on others or perhaps become very controlling and manipulative. Some adopt an aggressive manner and may shout or lose their temper on occasions, whereas others may shy away from difficult decisions and leave their team to their own devices.

13.1.1 Managers Who Are Prone to Getting Angry

If your manager starts shouting at you, do not sit and take it; however, whatever you do, do not shout back. Say that you are sorry about whatever it is but would rather wait and discuss the matter when things have calmed down. Say that you will leave if necessary. Only stay if they agree to talk to you in a civil manner. By saying that you prefer to wait until things have calmed down, it does not look like you are blaming them. You need to be diplomatic and it is important to remember that just because your manager, or anyone, is angry at you does not obligate you to become angry in return. Unfortunately, there are some managers who are continuously aggressive and intimidating. Explain that this approach of shouting at you is not going to make you work any harder. It just serves to upset and intimidate you. If you have made a mistake, always admit to it. If you have not done something that was asked for, state clearly and succinctly the reasons why you have not achieved what is required. Do not make excuses, which may only serve to increase their anger. If this is a situation that comes up time and time again, go and discuss it through with either your manager's line manager or someone senior in your human resources (HR) department. It is best to let your manager know first of your intentions. This may well stop the situation by itself. All NHS organisations are required to have a policy for dealing with bullying and harassment. You should be well supported through the process (although you must keep a factual log of all incidents as evidence).

13.1.2 Managers Who Do Not Manage

Some managers are reluctant to take on their managerial responsibilities. These tend to be people who are promoted because of their clinical experience. As mentioned previously, clinical skills are not the same as managerial skills. These types of managers may busy themselves with issues that require their clinical expertise and ignore their managerial role. It can be hard to get them to make any decisions or take any action on important managerial matters. It is difficult to deal with this sort of manager because they are normally well liked and maintain a good rapport with everyone. They will spend a lot of time sympathising with you and your team over your issues, but do not actually do anything about them. People tend to label them as 'supportive' managers because they spend time listening to individual problems (despite not doing anything about them). One way of dealing with this type of manager is to never present issues as problems, try and present the full solution to the problem, or a number of alternative solutions from which the manager can choose. For each solution, make sure

- it has been fully researched and meets the appropriate guidelines or policy;
- the appropriate people have been consulted;
- the implications have been considered in depth.

Bear in mind that these managers tend to thrive on social acceptance among the clinical team so ensure you make it clear that your solutions have been generated by your team and reflect all their views too.

13.1.3 Managers Who Expect Too Much

It can be hard for managers whose working day used to revolve around patients' needs to enter a world where it revolves around managing others. Patients' needs were always the priority, but when the next role no longer entails looking after patients, it can be difficult to work out what the priorities are. Some will take on too much work to compensate for this and over the years may get into a pattern of being very busy but not actually achieving anything. Some will take on extra projects or find it difficult to say no when bombarded with demands from their own senior managers. The problem for you is that some managers end up working extra long hours and you may find that some of this extra work is being delegated down to you. If this is happening and it gets too much (and you are certain that you are managing your own time effectively), then you must say so. Work out what your priorities and time commitments are (see Chapter 2), then go and discuss them with your manager. This can achieve two things:

1. Your manager will hopefully stop delegating the extra work to you.
2. Having seen what you have done, your manager may be stimulated into defining and prioritising their own workload using the same formula.

13.2 THE PROBLEMATIC COLLEAGUE

The very nature of our work means we will always be working with people, occasionally some very difficult people. Unfortunately, you cannot choose your work colleagues, and in the clinically focused role of the ward manager, you cannot retreat to an office or work alone to avoid the problem. So how do you handle a colleague who is proving rather difficult to work with? First, tell them. This sounds fairly obvious, but you would be amazed at how many do not do this. The individual then carries on blissfully unaware of the angst they are causing, and they are not doing it with malicious intent, despite the negative impact. By telling them, it is surprising how often the person will stop what they have doing, will apologise for any distress they have caused and will endeavour to not let it happen again. The situation will get worse if you leave it, and the longer you leave telling your colleague, the worse they will feel. Second, do not get personal, otherwise they will become defensive and you will get nowhere. Focus on the issue, not the person.

13.2.1 Colleagues Who Tend to Be Continually Negative and/or Complaining

Negative people are often insecure and unsure of themselves. By saying negative things about others, they are often trying to cover up their own limitations. Make an effort to share your ideas with them. Get them on your side by offering to take on some work together. Boost their confidence by giving them positive feedback on things they do well.

If you have a colleague who is always finding fault with people, ask what they have done or plan to do about the problem:

- What have you done about his/her behaviour?
- Have you told him/her how you feel?

The more often you question what they have done about it, the less they will find fault.

13.2.2 Colleagues Who Put Themselves Down All the Time

Colleagues who turn the criticism on themselves, saying things like 'I'm not good enough', are usually lacking in confidence. It is easier to criticise themselves before anyone else does. With a colleague like this, you can help simply by telling them that they are doing a good job and to stop talking themselves down. Those who put themselves down to receive compliments and praise from others are often also quite insecure. It is important to come to all of these people from a place of compassion as there are many number of reasons that they may be like this, including childhoods where there was not the validation and love you may take for granted. Take time with them and gently call out their behaviour to remind them of what they are doing and its impact on others.

13.2.3 Colleagues Who Are Continually Calling for Advice and Support

Some of your less experienced colleagues may have found you so helpful in the past that they continue to turn to you for every problem they encounter. If this happens, encourage them to seek a mentor/clinical supervisor for extra support. Tell them that relying on you alone for advice and guidance will restrict their learning; they have to seek support from others as well as you. Whenever this person calls you, always ask them first what they think is the best action and enable them to come to their own conclusions and actions.

13.3 ALLEGATIONS OF BULLYING OR HARASSMENT WITHIN YOUR TEAM

13.3.1 What Is Bullying or Harassment?

If members of your team do not treat their colleagues with dignity and respect, it could be interpreted as bullying or harassment. Situations in which a member of your team feels threatened, insulted or intimidated in any way by another person's behaviour must be stopped immediately. If any of your staff come to you saying that someone else makes them feel this way, even if it was not intended, you need to take action. If you do not do anything:

1. The individual's confidence and self-esteem will corrode and therefore affect their standard of work.
2. Other staff will get involved and begin to take sides, thus creating tension within the team.

Incivility and its more extreme cousins, bullying and harassment, have consequences. Porath and Pearson (2013) noted what happens when someone is rude:

80% of recipients lose time worrying about the rudeness.
38% reduce the quality of their work.
48% reduce their time at work.
25% take it out on service users.
For witnesses:
20% decrease in performance.
50% decrease in willingness to help others.

You should take all complaints seriously, even if you personally believe that it is simply a case of firm management or a harmless joke. Bullying and harassment are defined as any sort of behaviour which makes an individual feel upset, threatened, humiliated or vulnerable and undermines their confidence. In other words, it is the *impact* of the behaviour, not the *intent* of the perpetrator, which determines whether the person is being bullied or harassed.

Be aware that bullying can include the following:

- regular shouting or criticism in front of others
- refusing to speak to someone directly
- excessive supervision or checking up on a colleague's work
- constantly giving menial or trivial tasks to others
- deliberately excluding individuals from work-related social events
- unreasonably refusing requests for time off or training.

Harassment is any unwanted behaviour towards an individual regarding gender, race, disability, sexual orientation, religion, beliefs or any personal characteristic. This can include the following:

- intrusive questioning or gossiping about a person's private life, religion, activities, sexual orientation, etc.
- being condescending about the way a person dresses or speaks
- insensitive jokes or pranks
- unnecessary body contact

13.3.2 What Steps Should You Take?

When a member of staff complains to you that another person's behaviour is insulting or demeaning, your first step is to encourage them to tell the perpetrator, if they have not already done so. Sometimes people do not realise the effect they are having on others. Once informed, many will alter their behaviour. The individual who came to you may be low in confidence and therefore may need your support to do this. It is far better to work through with the individual what approach to take and encourage them to do it for themselves. This will increase their self-esteem and enable them to deal with any future situations with more confidence. However, the situation may be such that you will need to act as mediator between the two parties. In this case, make sure you have both parties present, otherwise you will get caught between two different versions of events and not know who to believe.

13.3.3 What Do You Do if Your Initial Approach Does Not Work?

If the perpetrator does not change their behaviour, you may have to intervene and use a more direct approach. In other words, tell the perpetrator to change their behaviour. If this does not work, the staff member at this stage can take a more formal approach by putting their concerns in writing. You should be liaising closely with your HR advisor throughout the process and ensuring that both parties involved in the allegation have access to support from their trade union representatives. Once a formal allegation is made, a manager from outside your ward will usually be brought in to undertake a formal investigation. This means that those involved, including you and other staff members, will be interviewed and statements taken. A report will be written with recommendations as to what actions should be taken. The recommended actions could include a number of things such as the following:

● an apology
● transfer of either party to another ward or department
● counselling or time off
● identification of training needs
● a disciplinary hearing up to and including dismissal and being reported to the NMC with a view to being struck off the register

Every NHS organisation is required to have a specific policy and guidelines for cases of bullying and harassment. It is wise to make yourself familiar with this policy. Also ensure your team are familiar with what your organisation defines as bullying and harassment. It will increase their awareness that bullying and harassment do not just concern people who shout and use violent threatening behaviour.

13.4 STAFF COMPLAINTS

Hopefully, you will have created a good healthy working atmosphere so that your team will be happy to bring issues to your attention if they have any concerns about their working conditions, standards of patient care or relationships with colleagues. Your leadership style should also ensure that all staff are willing to work together to agree some sort of solution. This includes taking the time to listen to their concerns and being willing to help them work through the issue and ensure something is done to resolve the situation.

13.4.1 Grievance Process

If people think of you as not particularly approachable or if any staff members are unhappy with your response to their concerns, they can raise a formal grievance. An individual grievance is a specific complaint from an individual against management and/or the Trust, concerning a matter related to their employment. A collective grievance is a specific complaint from a group of employees against management and/or the Trust, concerning a matter related to their employment, which those employees have agreed should be raised together.

Most employers have agreed grievance procedures which, to ensure a fair process is followed, should have at least three key stages:

1. the option to resolve the issue informally
2. the first formal stage
3. the opportunity to appeal the decision

If a grievance has been lodged against you as a manager, you should firstly seek advice and support from your HR department. When your employer discusses the allegations with you, be ready and able to justify any managerial decisions or actions you took in line with your employer's policies. At this initial stage, you are not being investigated or disciplined.

Generally, staff will only resort to this after they have exhausted all other options, which mainly consists of getting you to listen to them and take note of their concerns. All NHS organisations are required to have a grievance procedure, and it is usually strict in terms of the timetable to which you have to keep. If you receive a written complaint from a member of your staff about their working conditions, standards of care or relationships with colleagues, you should invite them to meet with you as soon as possible and inform them that they have a right to be accompanied by a friend, colleague or trade union representative as informal resolutions are where most grievances end. If the solution is outside your authority or if the grievance is against you personally, you should refer the matter to your line manager. Most policies state that you must have a meeting with them within a certain number of days from receipt of the letter; always check your local policy as it is normally a short time span. At this meeting you should do the following:

1. Allow the staff member to explain their complaint and what they think the solution should be.
2. Discuss and agree on a solution, or if you are not sure what to do about the complaint, you can then adjourn the meeting while you seek further advice.
3. Follow up the meeting with a letter confirming what was agreed. Your policy will state when this is to be done. It is usually within 3–5 days following the meeting.

13.4.2 What to Do if You Cannot Resolve the Complaint Alone

If the complaint is not resolved, the individual can write to your line manager who, in turn, can either meet with them to discuss the issue or send a written response. Again, your policy will set a time limit for the response, which is usually within 3–5 days from receipt of the letter. If your line manager cannot resolve the issue, the individual can then take it to the next managerial level. Again, they will either meet with the individual or write a letter. If the individual is still not satisfied, they can raise an appeal at board level. At this stage, one of the seniors will arrange an appeal panel. They will consider all the evidence including statements from any witnesses or representatives. The appeal panel decision is final.

13.5 Helping Your Staff to Act

You may be personally confident in dealing with difficult people when you are on duty, but part of your role is to ensure that your team are equipped with the skills to deal with difficult people and situations when you are not there.

13.5.1 The 'Difficult' Medical Consultant

Working partnerships between medical and nursing staff have not always been easy. Nowadays, on balance, things have changed significantly for the better. Nursing training is more academically focused, and nursing roles and responsibilities have expanded to include many of those previously done by junior doctors. The nursing profession nowadays is less hierarchical and more patient-centred. There are some consultants who still feel they are the ultimate boss and everyone should do as they say, and woe betide those who dare to question their decisions. These types are rare but still around and can be quite difficult to handle. Sometimes the arrogance is a cover-up for the fact that they do have a highly stressful job and may well suffer from inner feelings of insecurity about what they are doing. As Adam Kay's book *This is Going to Hurt: Secret Diaries of a Junior Doctor* (Kay 2017) revealed, the life of junior doctors especially still remains especially challenging with long hours, too often little support, exam pressures and a sense of isolation that means female doctors have a much higher risk of committing suicide compared with the general population Kinman & Teogh (2018).

How many times have you given a consultant any positive feedback on their work, or seen others do so? It can be quite an isolating role, especially for those who have had no training and development in communication or leadership skills. How do they know what they need? One way of dealing with this behaviour is to put extra effort into building up a good working relationship with them right from the start. Give positive feedback regularly and any negative feedback will be taken more seriously. If you only give negative feedback (i.e. keep telling them that their behaviour is unacceptable on your ward), they will assume that you are simply whingeing all the time. You will be seen as the problem, not them. Do not encourage your staff to confront them about their behaviour. Instead, show them by good role modelling how to talk to all consultants with confidence and how to give regular feedback. Include your staff in all areas of decision-making including ward rounds. Always encourage them to join in any discussions with your support rather than to be passive bystanders.

13.5.2 Bed Managers

Bed managers can never please everyone and it is probably one of the most difficult jobs in the NHS. Emergency department staff get fed up with them because patients are stacking up, ward staff are fed up with them for constantly pestering about the 'bed state' and discharges, managers are constantly pestering them to avoid target breaches; they get hassled from all sides. It is no wonder that they may pressurise your staff to discharge too early or to admit patients when they are not ready. When you are on duty, it should not be a problem. But what do you do if your staff are coerced into making decisions when you are not there; decisions that may not be appropriate such as taking extra or inappropriate patients into an already overstretched team of staff? It is difficult to refuse, especially if a matron or general manager becomes involved. If you find this has happened when you return from 'days off', the first thing to do is to speak to the bed manager as soon as you can to ascertain the facts. It is not unusual for staff to overstate their case a little when in reality they did little to explain their position to the bed manager. If you find out that members of your staff were forced into compromising patient care to meet targets, then explain to the bed manager that you are not happy and do not wish it to happen again in the future. Confirm the discussion plus your agreed actions briefly by email. Keep a file note of the conversation. This is usually enough to ensure it does not happen again. If it does happen again, do the same and involve more senior managers if necessary. The appropriate people must be made aware of what is happening. In the meantime, make sure that you set criteria with your team about bed decisions such as when to declare a bed is ready to take the next patient, that is, when the patient is no longer on the ward, or can wait in the dayroom only if they are fit and do not require any onerous nursing care or attention while there. Make sure the bed manager, matron and general manager are fully aware and involved in the development of these guidelines. Your organisation may already have some, so do not write new ones unless your ward or department is an exception.

13.5.3 Overloaded Link Nurses

Always be aware about what your link nurses are being asked to do. Their role is to act as a link between the nurse specialist or practice development team and the wards. These nurse specialists and practice development teams usually have a huge agenda and have goals to implement across the organisation. Often the only way they can communicate is through the link nurses. It is an effective system of disseminating information. Be supportive of them and be mindful of their workload, especially if they are unable to cope and/or start delegating it unfairly to members of your team. It is important you meet with them regularly to maintain good relations, boundaries and support.

13.6 DEALING WITH RACISM OR OTHER FORMS OF DISCRIMINATION

13.6.1 Patients and Relatives

One in five nurses generally and in some regions such as London up to two in five are from a BME background (Kline, 2014; NHS England and NHS Improvement, 2017). If a patient or relative refuses care because they object to the nurse's appearance, skin colour, religion, etc., despite the fact that the person is a competent nurse, then it should not be tolerated. This sounds simple but there are still recent examples in which healthcare professionals were not supported by their managers when discriminated against by patients or relatives. In 2004, a nurse was awarded £20,000 in compensation when a relative asked that she should not look after her baby because she was black. The manager moved the baby to another ward. In 2006, a nurse won a case of sex discrimination because he was not allowed to undertake procedures in his training such as ECGs on female patients without a chaperone. Moghal (2014) argues that simply transferring care to another clinician simply based on race is a form of institutional racism. If patients or relatives on your ward discriminate against your staff in any way, make sure you support them by telling the patient or relative that their comments are offensive. Remain polite and respectful. You will not be able to change the person's views, so it is not wise to attempt it. Just explain that their behaviour will not be tolerated. All members of your team should be assured privately and publicly that they will have your full support in any cases of this kind. Never dismiss any discriminatory comments as trivial and do not move the patient or nurse unless the nurse specifically requests not to look after them. If the patient or relative refuses care on discriminatory grounds, they should be made aware that they are effectively refusing services altogether. If the patient or relative will not listen to you or the nurse involved, consult your organisation's zero tolerance policy. All NHS organisations are required to have such a policy, which outlines what steps you can take when discriminatory behaviour persists after you have told them that it is unacceptable. The next step usually involves giving a written warning setting out types of behaviour that will no longer be tolerated. You do have a right to withdraw care but only with the backing of senior hospital managers.

13.6.2 Coworkers

Sadly, most racism experienced by nurses comes from coworkers rather than patients or senior managers (Kline, 2014; Das Gupta, 2009). It is quite clear within the Nursing and Midwifery Council (NMC) code that 'You must treat your colleagues fairly and without discrimination' (NMC, 2015). Filling the gaps in the health service with internationally sourced nurses has revealed some alarming discriminatory practices within the United Kingdom, and the results of the 2016 Brexit referendum to leave the European Union in 2019 have accentuated this in some places. These include questioning of competence, giving special negative attention if mistakes are made and stereotyping. This is more likely to be because the nurse is a foreigner or has a different cultural background than because of their colour or ethnicity. Take action to ensure this does not happen within your team. Your role as a manager is to give overseas nurses the same treatment as any other new recruit. However, you should bear in mind that having come from another country, it will take them longer to settle in and adapt to UK working practices.

1. *Prepare your team for their arrival.* Get your staff to think how they would feel starting a new job in a different country. It usually takes at least 3 months to settle in. Allow them to make mistakes without judging them negatively and ensure your team help them to learn from their experiences, including their mistakes.
2. *Ensure all new recruits have a minimum 2-week induction programme* (even if your organisation has already provided a programme specifically for the whole group of overseas nurses).
3. *Ensure each new nurse has at least one mentor* and that those mentors have attended awareness sessions on equality and diversity. Some organisations set up specific sessions for staff to learn about the culture of the country they have just recruited from.
4. *Make sure their personal development plan focuses on skills that they can transfer back home*, while ensuring they have the same career opportunities as the rest of your staff.
5. *Do not ever indulge in discussions* about 'the overseas nurses' where *they* are stereotyped by remarks such as 'good workers, never complain, a bit slow, not very assertive, etc.' Remember, no two individuals are the same, no matter what country they come from.

13.7 UNSAFE STAFFING LEVELS

13.7.1 Prioritise Patient Safety

Nurses, unlike many other professions, work to *minimum* safe staffing levels rather than *maximum* levels. Very few wards or departments are in a position where they can ever exceed their minimum staffing levels. This means that when someone goes off sick, you need bank or agency staff to cover. But there may be situations when

- more than one member of staff phones in sick
- there are not enough bank or agency staff to cover
- members of staff call in sick or are sent home during the course of a shift
- the workload suddenly and unexpectedly increases beyond your team's capacity to provide the required patient care

Most will be familiar with the following actions to take in such circumstances:

1. Inform a senior manager to see if staff can be moved from elsewhere in the hospital.
2. Phone/text around for staff to come in. Most wards and departments keep a list of staff home numbers, which will be used in such emergencies. (Remember that this is confidential information and must be kept locked away.)
3. Inform all relevant managers of the situation, including the bed manager, to ensure that patients are admitted elsewhere, and cancel any further admissions where possible.
4. Fill in an incident form.

Once every avenue has been attempted, some nurses forget the most important last step; to *prioritise*. If your workload is far greater than your capacity to deliver, do not tell your staff to just do what they can. That is tantamount to muddling through and is dangerous. Important things may be missed. Ensure your team take some time after handover to work out with their team what care is essential and what is desirable (i.e. can be left) for that shift. When very short staffed, maintaining the patients' safety becomes a greater priority than the provision of a high standard of care. Your team should be able to decide among themselves issues such as

- which patients need a full blanket bath and which patients can just make do with a hands and face wash;
- any administration that does not affect individual care such as audits and unnecessary form filling *will* be left undone.

These must be conscious decisions and not left to chance. Do not expect your staff to do everything as if normally staffed saying that it is fine if things get missed or mistakes get made. Short staffing is not an excuse for mistakes. Keep the patients and relatives informed and ensure the daily staffing notice of what numbers of staff you should have on duty and how many you actually have is in a prominent place. A notice such as this will make sure that your patients and their relatives are still confident in your management skills despite the fact that you are obviously short staffed.

13.7.2 Put Everything in Writing

Inform your line manager not only about the situation but also what you and your team have decided in terms of the care that is to be administered and which aspects of care will be left undone to maintain basic safe standards for all patients. Confirm the situation and the decisions that you made via an email to the appropriate manager. If the situation happens when you are not on duty, make sure your team know to take such actions, keep written notes and inform the appropriate people of their decisions. Try not to fill in the shift yourself each time unless absolutely necessary, and do not expect your staff to either. Part of your role as a manager is to ensure that your team are fit and well, and maintain a good work/life balance, not to work them to exhaustion. Your role is to look ahead and deal with the cause of the short staffing, not to continually 'plug the gaps'.

13.7.3 Incident Forms

You are usually required to fill in an incident form each time your team are subject to dangerously low staffing conditions. It is good to ensure that the situation is being noted, but incident reporting is not taking action; it is simply monitoring the situation. Do not just write who has been informed in the section entitled 'Action taken'. Write what action you have taken in terms of the priorities you have made with your team and your decisions about what will not be done. If the number of slips, trips and falls increases due to shorter levels of staffing, you will be able to prove via the incident forms that you have done everything in your power to prevent this.

13.8 CLIQUES

Despite your best intentions, you may find that cliques form within your team, particularly if you have members of staff who have been with you for many years. These long-term employees can be invaluable in terms of stability and maintaining high standards. They tend to be loyal and can become almost like part of a family. However, it can have a detrimental effect, especially with newcomers to the team who find it difficult to fit in.

13.8.1 Effects on New Recruits

Cliques can result in the loss of self-confidence of a new member of staff. Their work may suffer and you could find you have a new staff nurse who is not quite living up to your initial expectations. Worse still, they may leave within a few months for another job but not tell you the real reason; in fact, they may not realise the reason themselves. If someone does not fit in to a new work environment, they tend to blame themselves for not having the right social skills. Few may admit that to their manager, so you will be left in the dark as to the real reason. Try and be alert to the signs.

13.8.2 Breaking Up a Clique in Your Team

Cliques that are causing problems within your team need to be broken up. There are several ways you can do this. The first and most obvious is to arrange the roster so that they do not always work together. When they are on duty together, encourage them to take different breaks as much as possible. Another option is to select one or two members of the clique and give them specific tasks or projects for which they must report to you. Give them lots of encouragement, praise and rewards for a job well done. A similar result may be gained if you ensure that each time you recruit a new member of staff, you assign one member of the clique to be their mentor. Give the mentor lots of positive feedback around their work with the newcomer.

13.8.3 Promotion to Ward Manager Within the Same Team

You may find that when you become a ward manager it could well be on the same ward where you have been in a senior staff nurse or deputy ward manager role and you have done so with skills as a clinician that support your ability to lead a team (NHS Improvement, 2018). You will be in the unenviable position of managing staff whom you have been working alongside very well for some time. You may find that they are happy with the situation and continue to work well as a team. However, be mindful of new members coming into the team; you could unwittingly become part of a clique. This happens so easily. So, if your first ward manager's post is on the same ward with the same team, it is advisable to take the following actions (Thomas and Osborne-McKenzie, 2018):

1. Meet one-on-one with each member of the team. By having your first manager-team member conversations individually, you will be able to personalise the message and be more candid than you can be in a group setting. Ask questions like 'are there any specific areas where you like my support?' Listen carefully, be respectful and it will help your team realise you have not suddenly become a power-crazy manager!
2. Do share your vision for the unit and the team and ask for feedback so your team can own it too.
3. There is no need to pretend you suddenly have all the answers. They were your peers before appointment and know you well. Ask for support, especially where any of them have particular skills you lack or are still building.
4. At the first team meeting, bring in some of the ideas from the one-on-one meetings you have had and reiterate them. Discuss the goals of the team and how they can be achieved together.
5. Articulate how you like to work and share some of your own philosophy. Encourage questions and ideally, do something social afterwards so there is recognition that you are still you even if your role has changed. One thing that may need to occur is your behaviour will be watched even more closely now so there needs to be modelling of both your espoused and lived personal and professional behaviours.

13.8.4 What if Your Own Line Manager Is Part of a Clique?

You may find yourself in a situation where you are managing a team that has worked together for years and which includes your own line manager. They may even have trained together. This is not an uncommon situation, but you must take control of it. Do not let your position be undermined by letting your staff bypass you and going to your line manager, who also happens to be an old friend of theirs, about issues pertaining to your ward. If your line manager is taking time to listen to your staff concerns and starting to intervene without involving you, tell them how damaging the situation is. They may think that they are helping you out by listening to their friends/old colleagues and reporting back to you, but this can be more of a hindrance than a help. Agree on a joint strategy with your line manager about what action you would prefer to be taken when a member of your team goes to them; that is, refer that person back to you and do not take the time to listen to the concerns until that staff member has spoken with you first. If your line manager allows the clique to continue and you find them liaising with your team and not involving you, you could try explaining the situation to their line manager and asking for their intervention. Whatever you do, do not let the situation continue. It can gradually erode your confidence in your ward management skills and could be quite damaging for team morale.

13.9 BE SPECIFIC ABOUT EXPANDING NURSING ROLES

Expanding roles is an area where as a manager you need to be proactive. It is not advisable to allow some staff to take on extra roles and other staff not to, because this can cause great divisions within your team. One example is intravenous cannulation and venepuncture. If you allow your nurses individually to decide whether or not to undertake training, you may find that

- those nurses who can cannulate and take blood have to undertake it for all the patients and not just their own;
- doctors may resent the nurses who do not cannulate or take blood and will be less willing to undertake what they come to see as the nurses' role;
- the nurses who do not cannulate or take blood may resent those who do, because they feel they are doing doctors work and not their own;
- patients will see nurses that do not cannulate or take blood as less experienced.

Before you take on an extra role to be taken on in your area, discuss it as a team first. Go through the advantages and disadvantages of the added responsibility. Decide together as a team whether to embrace the new role or reject it. It you decide to embrace it, then all members of the team must train and use the skills in practice. The NMC (2018) standards framework for nursing and midwifery education offers very helpful guidance on the standards expected of approved education institutions delivering content for nursing practice.

13.10 BE PROACTIVE WITH ENFORCED MOVES OR MERGERS OF SERVICES

It is widely recognised that to successfully reorganise, all staff should be given the opportunity to contribute and be involved in the changes. In other words, if your ward or department needs to be moved, merged or restructured in any way, your managers should ensure that you and your staff are fully consulted and involved in making that decision, including the consideration of all alternatives.

13.10.1 Get Involved

You may find that you were not involved in making the decision. Some senior managers focus more on the outcome than the process, of which communication and staff involvement are a great part. However, do not always blame the hospital board of directors or your managers if decisions are made without your involvement. If you are making full use of your networking and political awareness skills, you will probably have ensured your involvement to some extent.

13.10.2 Plan ahead

If you find that your service is going to be restructured, you must plan ahead for this change. Even a relatively small change like moving your team to a different ward or site or merging with another team can result in long-lasting problems if not handled correctly. Staff morale can be affected, people will look elsewhere for jobs and the standard of care may well fall. First, find out why the restructuring is required and explain the facts to your team. Take care not to procrastinate, backbite or talk negatively about the decision in front of your team. If you disagree with the enforced change, make your feelings known to your managers but only if you can offer a realistic alternative solution. If you cannot, you will have to accept the decision and then focus on your main objectives, which are as follows:

- supporting, involving and developing your team;
- maintaining a good standard of patient care.

Develop a project plan with your team to manage the move or merger working with more senior managers. Only you and your staff will be able to identify and plan the finer details. Present the final project plan to your manager or, better still, involve your manager in the development of the plan.

13.10.3 Developing a Project Plan

So how do you develop a project plan? The following steps will help you in the process:

1. Find out what your deadline is for completing the move or merger.
2. Inform your team as soon as possible. Take time to listen to their concerns and explain why the decision has been made. Make sure all valid concerns are relayed back to your manager in writing.

3. Visit the area you are moving to or meet the manager of the team you will be merging with.
4. Hold a team meeting for your staff in which you
   a. brainstorm with all your team what issues need to be considered (e.g. equipment, extra skills that staff may need) and define the tasks that need to be undertaken;
   b. break up the tasks into different phases, usually in terms of weeks (e.g. week 1, week 2, week 3, etc.);
   c. compile a simple Gantt chart (see Appendix 13.1);
   d. for each task, determine what needs to be done and by whom.
      If you are merging with another team, hold the above meeting with both teams together.
5. Set dates for regular review meetings with the team to review progress against the Gantt chart and identify any problems or issues that need further attention.
   Always remember that you can never communicate enough in such situations. With a team covering 24 h per day, 7 days per week, you cannot communicate through team meetings alone. Use every other method open to you such as the ward communication book, handovers, staff notice board, etc.

13.10.4 Involve the Experts From the Beginning

Involve your finance manager in all stages of the plan to ensure that staff time and resources are appropriately costed and accounted for. Extra funding is usually allocated to assist with any move or merger; make sure that it is appropriately utilised. Involve your HR manager early if staff roles are changing. They will advise on the appropriate consultation and involvement of union representatives. Do not leave all this to your manager, who will themselves likely be intensely busy already, as you are the best person to lead the process. You understand the needs of your staff and patients better than anyone else. Your manager's role is to help, support and guide you through the process.

13.10.5 Action Points

- If you have difficulties with your manager, start thinking about the situation from their perspective and take positive steps to improve your working relationship.
- Read through your organisation's bullying and harassment policy and familiarise yourself with what is classed as 'unacceptable behaviour'.
- Take all staff complaints seriously to avoid the need for formal grievances to be made. If a formal grievance is made, read the policy and take action quickly to remain within the tight timescales of the policy.

- Concentrate on developing the skills of your staff to deal with problematic senior healthcare professionals.
- Be aware and deal appropriately with any forms of discrimination, particularly towards your staff from patients, relatives or other members of your team.
- Ensure your team are aware of their responsibilities regarding equality and diversity.
- Make sure your staff formally prioritise and make sure their decisions are relayed to the appropriate line manager in writing when staffing levels are unsafe.
- Break up cliques using the roster and allocating members of the clique to orientate new recruits. Devise a joint strategy with your own line manager to break up a clique if your line manager is involved.
- Decide jointly with your staff which expanded nursing roles you will all undertake, ensuring the appropriate training and guidelines are available.
- Develop a project plan and Gantt chart with your team to help deal with any major changes, such as a ward move or merger.
- Do not ignore problematic colleagues. Take appropriate action now.

APPENDIX 13.1 EXAMPLE OF SIMPLE GANTT CHART FOR WARD MOVE/MERGER

Actions	Week No.							
	1	2	3	4	5	6	7	8
1. Equipment								
Compile equipment inventory			→					
Sort and label each piece						→		
2. Staffing								
Meet staff to clarify position	→							
Identify skills deficit			→					
Training and development							→	
3. Review progress								
Meetings with whole team	×		×		×		×	
4. Documentation								
Gather all from both units	→							
Consult both teams		→						
Agree on best practice			→					
Communicate to all teams				→				
Sort out ordering process						→		
5. Guidelines and policies								
Identify all policies		→						
Set subgroups to merge			→					
6. Moving patients								
Agree plan with bed manager						→		
Stop admitting patients							→	
Transfer remaining patients								→

REFERENCES

Clarke, R., McKee, M., 2018. Suicides among junior doctors in the NHS. British Medical Journal 357.

Das Gupta, T., 2009. Real Nurses and Others: Racism in Nursing. Fernwood Press, Halifax.

Kay, A., 2017. This Is Going to Hurt: Secret Diaries of a Junior Doctor. Picador, London.

Kinman, G., Teoh, K., 2018. What Could Make a Difference to the Mental Health of UK Doctors? Society of Occupational Medicine.

Kline, R., 2014. The 'Snowy White Peaks' of the NHS: A Survey of Discrimination in Governance and Leadership and the Potential Impact on Patient Care in London and England. Middlesex University, London.

Moghal, N., 2014. Allowing patients to choose the ethnicity of attending doctors is institutional racism.

NHS England, NHS Improvement, 2017. Enabling BME Nurse and Midwife Progression into Senior Leadership. NHSE/NHSI, London.

NHS Improvement, 2018a. The Ward Leaders Handbook. NHS Improvement, London.

NHS Improvement, 2018b. Developing Workforce Safeguards: Supporting Providers to Deliver High Quality Care through Safe and Effective Staffing. NHS Improvement, London.

Nursing and Midwifery Council, 2015. The Code: Professional Standards of Practice and Behaviour for Nurses and Midwives. NMC, London.

Nursing and Midwifery Council, 2018. Realising Professionalism: Standards for Education and Training. Part 1: Standards Framework for Nursing and Midwifery Education. NMC, London.

Pearson, C., Porath, C., 2009. The Cost of Bad Behaviour: How Incivility is Damaging Your Business and What to do About it. Penguin, New York.

Thomas, J., Osborne-McKenzie, T., 2018. From buddy to boss: transitioning from 'one of us' to 'one of them'. Nurse Leader 315–318.

Chapter 14

Manage Difficult Team Members

If you are having problems dealing with inappropriate behaviour from members of your team, you need to look first at your style of leadership. Have you established team objectives? Are you really listening to your team and providing them with regular feedback on their performance? Do you know them well and do you spend time enhancing their individual strengths within the team? If not, go back to Chapter 3 and review your own leadership style before you focus on dealing with the individual problems.

However, even with the best of leadership skills, there may be the occasional instance when individuals in your team do behave in an unacceptable manner. These situations need to be dealt with swiftly. Be clear of your standards. Do not avoid the situation and do not let the individual(s) avoid you. The rest of the team will be watching you to see what you do. They will not respect a leader who ignores episodes of inappropriate behaviour.

14.1 STAFF WHO REFUSE TO LOOK PROFESSIONAL OR WEAR PROPER UNIFORM

If members of your team are deliberately flouting the uniform policy or dress code, it can be a sign of rebelliousness. Think first and foremost, 'Is there any reason why they may wish to rebel against you?' Disobedient behaviour is usually triggered when an individual feels that:

- they are not listened to
- they have no 'voice'
- their work is not fulfilling
- they have a controlling manager

If you have shared objectives, listen and give regular feedback and know your staff well, there should be little reason for individuals to want to rebel (see Chapter 3). But if you are having problems despite these measures, it is advisable to take action before the rest of the team follow suit and also start flouting the uniform policy. Staff members who refuse to dress appropriately for the job may be feeling unable to express themselves in any other way.

So, what do you do? First, do not just tell them what the dress code is; you can be fairly certain they will know what the policy entails. The best way to approach them is to ask about their behaviour. There will always be an underlying reason. Getting that reason to the surface depends on your questioning and listening abilities:

- 'Why are you wearing trainers/jewellery?'
- 'Why have you stopped tying your hair up?'

You may find you open a can of worms with answers such as:

- 'I do not feel we should be dictated to as to what we wear'.
- 'We are not at school anymore, and I object to being treated like a child'.

These sorts of answers should be explored with further questioning. A simple 'please help me understand why you feel like that?' would suffice. They may wish to make a statement, so allow them to make it. Empathise with their predicament and support them to take action in another way.

Explain the rationale behind the policy, and the effects that their behaviour may be having on patients and others, such as decreasing people's confidence in their skills, patients' health and safety being compromised or exposing vulnerable people to an increased risk of infection.

14.1.1 Is It an Individual Issue?

If there is only one individual involved, make sure the discussion is held in private. People who want to make a statement may feel they have won if they feel that others have taken notice, or that they have got something in return for behaving this way. Once you have listened to their issue, agree on appropriate alternative action and ensure they agree to abide by the terms of the policy in future. Make sure they are aware that if they continually breach the uniform policy or dress code, they are liable to disciplinary action. Remember to let them know that you will be making a file note of the discussion and agreed actions (see Chapter 4).

14.1.2 Is It a Team Issue?

If you have recently taken over a new team as a ward manager, you may find yourself confronted with several members or even the whole team who are not adhering to the uniform policy. It can be a tricky situation if they have been doing this for years. It would be advisable in such a situation to raise the issue at a team meeting and have a general discussion about dress codes and uniform issues.

14.1.3 Cultural, Race and Religious Requirements

While all staff should adhere to the uniform policy, you must be sensitive to the needs of different cultures, ethnicities and religions. You should be able to accommodate these needs within the uniform policy. If there are particular difficulties, consult your human resources (HR) advisor. It would not be appropriate to discipline staff for non-compliance from having to adhere to a particular cultural, race or religious dress code.

14.2 STAFF WHO REFUSE TO ACCEPT CHANGE

Some staff members can be rather obstinate when you want to change something at work. Remember that most people do not like change for its own sake and we often like to keep the status quo. In the majority of cases, people who refuse to change are doing so because they have not been consulted or involved in identifying the need for the change. Keeping your team fully *informed* at each stage is not sufficient; they must be fully *involved* at each stage of the process.

If, for example, you wish to implement bedside handover where previously you have been using the office only, you cannot expect your staff to simply conform even if you have explained your rationale and the advantages many times over. The key to implementing something like this effectively is to start right at the beginning by analysing the original problem with your team. In other words, get them together and look at what is wrong with the current system before you start suggesting the solution. Bedside handover is a solution. Do the team have a problem with the office handover? If so, what do they suggest should be done? Everyone will have different views; they must be listened to. If you do come to an agreement to think about a change such as bedside handover, it is a good idea to explore the concept first with your team. SWOT analysis is a common tool used in healthcare for analysing the need for change within a team.

14.2.1 SWOT Analysis

SWOT stands for 'strengths, weaknesses, opportunities and threats'.
Draw a matrix (Fig. 14.1) and get your team to identify:

- the strengths and weaknesses of your current system (internal)
- the opportunities and threats which may affect any future system (external)

Appendix 14.1 gives an example of a SWOT analysis. This tool helps teams to identify the weaknesses and threats of either the current system or the new

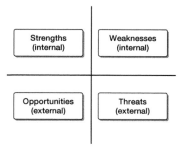

FIGURE 14.1   SWOT analysis.

system being proposed. But do not leave it there; otherwise you will just be left with a long list of factors and no attempt to do anything about it.

14.2.1.1 Getting Your Team to 'Own' the Solution

Your next step is to identify with the team what can be done to overcome the weaknesses and threats and make the most of your strengths and forthcoming opportunities. Only when you have all reached an agreement about what needs to be done should you begin the process of planning and implementing the change. Doing it this way round will reduce the chances of staff refusing to change. If anyone does not want to change, they should be encouraged to come up with a valid alternative solution. You should have given them ample opportunity to do this at your initial meeting.

Remember to make sure that all members of your team have the opportunity to take part. Keep notes of the meeting and make sure everyone gets to see them.

14.3 STAFF WHO CANNOT SEEM TO PRIORITISE THEIR WORK

Some staff will continually stay late in order to:

- complete their evaluations/notes
- finish off a task that could easily be delegated to someone else
- see to other patients whom they have neglected by concentrating on giving a high standard of care to a select few patients

People like this tend to be perfectionists and may lose track of time and priorities by continually striving to maintain high standards of care. However, with higher patient turnover, increasingly complex care requirements and continual staff shortages, maintaining exceptionally high standards of care all the time is not always realistic. If you allow them to continue striving to achieve these exceptionally high standards, it will result in either:

1. them becoming exhausted and ending up going off sick or leaving or
2. some patients receiving exceptionally high standards of care at the expense of others

14.3.1 Getting Staff to Manage Their Time More Effectively

Teaching people to manage their time at work becomes a lot more complex where unpredictable patient care is involved. A more effective method of helping this individual would be to take some time to work alongside them, preferably for whole shifts at a time. That way you (or one of the more senior members of your team) can help them recognise how to prioritise their work and how to deal with the unpredictable. Your seniority will also give them permission to lower their standards when necessary, such as in times of staff shortages. An example is helping a patient with partial paralysis from a recent stroke to get dressed. A high standard of care would be:

- to encourage the patient to do things for themselves throughout the process
- to spend time talking through the techniques they use, giving positive feedback and corrections where necessary
- to discuss any worries or concerns they may have
- to only physically intervene when absolutely necessary

However, rehabilitation takes a lot of time and patience. If the nurse has eight patients in a similar position, delivering an exceptionally high standard of care for every one of them may simply not be feasible within the time limits of their shift. They can either give all eight an acceptable standard of care, by talking the patient through some of the process and physically helping them through the rest, or purposefully delaying some parts of their care until the later shift comes on duty. It is also important to encourage the staff to engage with family members as they (and patients) are often under-utilised as a source of great care and in any case will be doing a lot of the care once the patient has left hospital.

14.3.2 Prevent Burnout

Many nurses have learnt how to manage their time and priorities through experience, but some are reluctant to lower their standards and end up exhausted by not taking their breaks or staying on late to finish their work. People who work like this rarely complain. They simply get on with it, thinking that they have to make sacrifices in order to deliver a high standard of care. Watch for people like this and take action before you end up with an exhausted and stressed member of staff. Often it is their home life and self-esteem that suffers long before the stress and exhaustion become an issue at work. By the time they reach the stage of taking time off sick from 'burnout', it may be too late for you to take action.

By spending time working with the individual as outlined above, you can show them how to work out which aspects of their work are the real priorities, and which are their own personal priorities. You cannot just tell people how to plan and prioritise their care at the beginning of the shift; things always change. A patient's condition may unexpectedly deteriorate or there may be unexpected admissions or transfers. If you work the whole shift with them, you can demonstrate how to re-prioritise as changes occur.

14.3.3 Maintaining Good Standards of Care

While it is advisable to ensure staff do not exhaust themselves maintaining unrealistically high standards, do not become too complacent about lowering standards of care to fit in with increasing demand. It should not come to be seen as normal practice. If your workload is increasing, make sure you are doing something about getting more staff added to your establishment to deal with the extra work, or working differently by applying lean methodologies to identify waste and eliminating them. A simple example is ensuring observation machines are returned to the same place after use so that staff are not wasting time wandering from bay to bay looking for them thus wasting time and adding to their sense of 'busyness'.

If staffing shortages are becoming a regular occurrence, you should be working closely with your manager to either find ways of changing or reducing the workload or increasing your staffing levels. You cannot sustain high workload with low staffing levels for any length of time without reducing standards and safety.

14.4 STAFF LABELLED AS LAZY

People may slip into what appear to be 'lazy' habits when they see their work as boring or unrewarding. They may slow down at work, perpetuate gossip and spend time on less important tasks rather than the ones that really matter.

People who are labelled as 'lazy' appear to be getting away with doing as little work as possible. This is usually because of one of three things:

1. Lethargy due to physical or mental illness,
2. Heavy personal life/non-work commitments,
3. Lack of motivation.

Before you take action, try and identify which one of the three it is. If the laziness is intermittent, then it may be because they lack motivation. If it is a permanent feature, there may be an underlying cause, such as illness. If it is because of poor physical or mental health (e.g. stress, depression or a long-term back problem), consider a GP referral, or a referral to the occupational health department for advice. Some time off sick may be all that is needed to recuperate.

If there are difficulties juggling family commitments with work, find out what you can do to facilitate adapting working hours around family life, such as:

- more flexible shift patterns
- different start and finish times
- temporary reduction in working hours

You may feel that the family life of staff members is their own problem, but such an attitude is unwise and it is far better to start from a place of compassion rather than judgement. Your role as a manager is to enable your team to provide their best efforts. Give less to your team and your team will give less to you. Whatever you do, you cannot ignore this issue with individual members of staff. It could lead to resentment from the rest of your team.

On the other hand, if a staff member thinks nothing of going out 'clubbing' between late and early shifts, they obviously do not value or appreciate their responsibilities as part of your team. This may well be a sign that they lack motivation at work. It can also be a patient safety issue as tired staff are more likely to make mistakes.

14.4.1 Dealing With Those Who Lack Motivation

People who are lazy for reasons other than illness or overwhelming personal responsibilities have discovered a way of not doing something that they do not want to do. Spending time talking to someone or persistently 'telling them off' because of their perceived laziness generally does not help. Their experience shows them that doing more is not in their best interests, so why should they change? The rewards for doing less work are probably far more preferable to the consequences of being reprimanded.

Find out how you can motivate them: it is all part of being a good leader – knowing what makes each individual in your team tick and taking time to work on those motivators (see p. 50). The unfortunate thing about managing people in healthcare is that you cannot provide monetary rewards, but there are other ways. Giving good feedback in front of others helps. Find out what part of their role they like and ensure they get to do this part only if they complete the 'boring' part. Reward-based systems have their place.

This is all about work/life balance. Whether the person is working too hard or playing too hard, the critical thing for you as their manager is to get them to re-evaluate and redress the imbalance.

14.4.2 Are They in the Right Job?

If a member of your staff cannot summon up any enthusiasm at all for their job, then it might be best to encourage them to consider whether this is the right job for them. If the work in your ward is not stimulating for them, despite your best efforts, then perhaps they are working in the wrong environment. Do not take this personally. Work with them to find out where their skills lie and what they really want to do, then help them towards that goal. Help to provide them with the appropriate training and development for their chosen role, and provide assistance with job applications, interviews and references on condition that they pull their weight at work in the meantime. At the very least, you are providing them with the required motivation to stop being lazy while they remain with you looking for another job.

14.5 STAFF WITH ALCOHOL PROBLEMS

14.5.1 Staff Who Turn up for Duty Drunk

What do you do when a member of staff turns up for duty who is obviously under the influence of alcohol? The answer is simple: send them home again. This can only be done by someone who is the person's direct line manager. If you are not on duty, the nurse-in-charge should consult with your line manager or whoever is on call. That manager will then make the decision to send the staff member home. There is usually no need to suspend the member of staff from duty or prevent their return the next day or when their next shift is due. Suspension of staff is only required if there is a risk of potential harm to patients or staff (or themselves).

The next step is up to you. For example, if this was a one-off incident and the member of staff is a competent worker with a previously unblemished record, you may decide to end the matter with a conversation about expected professional standards on their return and then informally monitor for any subsequent lapses in behaviour.

If you decide to follow the formal policy route, you should instigate a formal investigation into the incident. This is often done by an HR advisor, but could be anyone who is unrelated to the incident. They will interview all witnesses and formal statements will be taken. The staff member who was sent home will also be interviewed as part of the investigatory process. This gives them a chance to give their side of the story. Remember to ensure that any members of staff who are interviewed and required to give formal statements are informed of their rights to have a trade union representative, colleague or friend present.

The person appointed to carry out the investigation will gather all the evidence together in the form of a report and make recommendations. It all needs to be done as soon as possible after the event. The recommended action will depend on whether it is the individual's first offence (usually a verbal or written warning) or whether their actions were serious and detrimental to patient care (written warning or dismissal).

14.5.1.1 If It Is Not the First Offence or the Offence Is of a More Serious Nature

If this is not the first time that this has happened, or the person's actions were serious and detrimental to patient care, then you should follow the policy route. The investigation report may recommend a disciplinary hearing. It may also recommend that you provide further support or help for the person's drinking/personal problems. Your manager will make that decision and will lead the disciplinary panel where they will have the option to issue a formal verbal or written warning. If the circumstances surrounding the incident were very serious and compromised patient care, your manager could make a decision to dismiss at the disciplinary hearing with potential for referral to the NMC.

14.5.1.2 Staff Who Have a Long-Term Drinking or Drug Problem

Managing substandard work or misconduct due to prolonged alcoholism or drug misuse is an entirely different process and is generally treated as a health problem rather than an immediate cause for disciplinary action, although this may eventually be required.

You usually have the option of using any one of the three following procedures, depending on the circumstances:

1. Disciplinary procedure.
2. Capability or competency procedure.
3. Sickness/absence procedure.

There will also be a drugs/alcohol policy that you would need to refer to. Always consult your HR advisor, who will guide you as to which policy is most appropriate.

You should offer reasonable support if any members of staff admit that they have a problem with alcohol and/or drugs and who are prepared to make a concerted effort to overcome this. Your role is to treat these staff with sympathy and in complete confidence. Make sure you involve the occupational health department at an early stage. Part of your support process should include the granting of leave to see their GP or attend counselling sessions. Such action will be considered in the event of disciplinary action but will not be seen as an alternative to disciplinary action if it is deemed necessary.

In any event, be aware that your prime concern is the protection of the patients. If any registered nurse fails in their duty of care towards their patients due to the influence of alcohol and/or, you can dismiss them at a disciplinary hearing and you may also be obliged to recommend their removal from the register.

14.6 MEMBERS OF STAFF WHO DO NOT GET ON

Allowing personal differences to get in the way of work is unprofessional and should not be condoned. Since you are the one who is responsible for creating the right environment for good teamwork, you have a big role to play when members of your team do not get on as if left unattended, the situation can end up affecting the whole team. You must step in at once or other members of the team will begin choosing sides. Those not caught up in the conflict will look to you to resolve it.

Five suggested steps to resolving conflict within your team immediately are the following:

1. Bring the two team members into your office to work together on some sort of solution. Give them 5–10 min each to explain their position. They need to know that you have given them the chance to air their grievances. You are there as a manager, not a counsellor. Do not let them interrupt each other, find fault or try to apportion blame.
2. Once they have explained their sides, ask each in turn to say what they feel the other person should do differently. Make sure their solutions are clear and 'doable'. Something like 'I want her to change her attitude' is too general and does not get you anywhere. Get them to be more specific; get them to say exactly what they want the other person to stop doing, such as

'I want her to stop pulling a face and walking off whenever I ask her to help me with something'. Then get each in turn to say what they want the other person to do instead, such as 'I want her to tell me straight if she is unhappy with what I have asked her to do and why'.

3. When these actions have been clarified, get each side to commit to doing at least one of the suggested solutions. Get them to agree to give each other feedback and acknowledge times when the other person has made the effort to change. This gets both parties to focus on the positive side of things.

4. Let them know in plain terms that it is down to them to make this work. If they do not make the effort and allow the situation to continue, inform them that you will have no choice but to take formal action.

5. Make a brief file note of the discussion, including an outline of the agreed actions. Let them read it through and sign if necessary. Give each of them a copy.

Following this discussion, make it a priority to observe them closely over the next few weeks. Give positive feedback when you notice a change in their behaviour. Hopefully the situation will resolve. However, if it does not improve within a few weeks (do not leave it any longer), bring them both into your office again and outline the formal route that you will take should you see no improvement over the next couple of weeks. Again, make another file note.

Hopefully, the situation will be resolved following the second meeting. But if it is not, you will have no choice but to take the formal route. This is usually the disciplinary policy, but check first with your HR advisor, who will point you in the direction of any other appropriate policy that you may have within your organisation.

14.7 STAFF WHO SEEM CARELESS AND SLOPPY

It can be really frustrating when dealing with members of staff who do not give enough attention to the important details when caring for patients. Their work may be hurried and sloppy, but they may seem quite content and think that they are doing fine. Some people tend to make lots of mistakes but do not seem to see it as a problem. Important observations may not be done, discharge arrangements will be left for the next shift or patients requiring rehabilitation will be washed and dressed with no attention paid to assisting them to help themselves. They seem to find paying attention to detail as tiresome and dull.

One of the problems with having someone like this in your team is that it can cause resentment among the rest of the staff who constantly have to pick up the pieces. If you do not do anything about it, you are effectively sanctioning their behaviour. They could be perfectly happy to continue, while thinking that the rest of the team are at fault for making such a fuss.

14.7.1 Use of Competency Packages

Usually these types of people need to be told to slow down and take more responsibility for their patient care. You have to reiterate what the expected standards are. However, just saying this may not be sufficient. If the member of staff is junior and inexperienced, it may be a simple case of allocating a mentor to work through a competency package with them.

If the individual in question is more senior and experienced, why not get them to *develop* competences or *review* the competency package that you already have in place. Make sure that the areas of care being overlooked are included in the package. For example, if your area cares for patients requiring rehabilitation, do the competences specify how to assist the patients to help themselves rather than do everything for them? Does it assess the person's knowledge of when and why observations should be carried out? Does it set out each stage of the discharge process that should be covered and when?

Helping to write these standards down in the form of competences usually helps to stimulate the member of staff about the quality of care they are expected to provide rather than what they have got away with over the years. You may prefer to do this as part of a team meeting or discussion to help raise standards generally across the team.

14.7.2 Use of Positive Feedback to Enhance Good Behaviour

Reward the individual for when they have paid attention to detail by giving frequent positive feedback. When the work has not been done, get them to go back and correct or finish their work where possible. They need to learn that there are consequences for not producing an adequate standard of work.

Be prepared to stick at it. Members of staff who are careless and sloppy in their work will not change overnight. They have to unlearn their habits and acquire new ones, which takes time. If, after 3–6 months, you find that they have really not changed their ways, you should question their capability for undertaking the role. Most organisations have a policy which guides you through a specific process consisting of meetings and action plans to improve a person's capability (see Chapter 4). Ultimately, if you follow this policy, your manager could make the decision to terminate their employment if the process is unsuccessful, but you must have explored all other avenues first and kept a full record of all your actions in the form of file notes.

14.8 STAFF WHO MANIPULATE SITUATIONS FOR THEIR OWN GAIN

Some members of staff like to get their own way. This behaviour often becomes apparent when it has something to do with requests and the roster. There are some members of staff who do not care what effect their requests have on other staff. You may be familiar with excuses such as:

'You told me if I put the request in first then I could have it'.

'You promised me last year that I could have this weekend off'.

'I spoke to HR and they said that I could take 4 weeks' annual leave together and that you cannot refuse to give it to me'.

Manipulators will often play off one person against the other. They will go to more senior people if they cannot get their own way. This is particularly rife if individuals are aware that you and your manager do not communicate well or have any differences. Prevent this by ensuring that you never let staff know if there are problems between you and anyone else within your organisation. Manipulators are constantly on the lookout for these and will take advantage of any perceived breakdown in communications between you and your colleagues. Do not give them the opportunity. It is crucial to be seen as fair and even-handed with all members of staff.

14.8.1 Confront Them Directly

Often the only way to deal with these people is to confront them directly. Tell them exactly what you think is going on; the chances are that they will be taken by surprise. Many people who do this do it as a way of life and are unaware that their behaviour might be determined as manipulation. Explain that if they had taken a more straightforward approach, and simply asked you rather than going to someone else, they could have got what they wanted without any hassle. However, as they have now gone to someone else to try and override your authority, you are seeing things in a different light and are reluctant to concede to their demands. Tell them in future they must be more direct in their approach.

Another way is to meet with the other person whom they used to try and manipulate you. Explain the situation to them and ask the manipulator to meet with you both and explain their actions, and perhaps even apologise. Remember to acknowledge or give positive feedback in the future each time they do use a more direct approach for something they want.

14.8.2 Laying the Blame on You

With the ever-increasing emphasis on accountability within healthcare, you may find that some staff are reluctant to take responsibility for their mistakes. You may hear phrases such as:

'The band six said I could do this'.

'You told us that it did not matter if we did not do all the observations when it was busy'.

'It was not my fault. If you had not agreed to admit those extra patients, this would never have happened'.

In situations such as these, do not be tempted to go into defensive mode with replies such as:

'I did not say that'.
'When I said that I did not mean for you to go ahead and do this'.
'It is not my fault either; do not blame me'.

Do not get into a discussion about who is to blame: concentrate on what is to be done about the situation. Get people to focus on generating solutions. Then once the problem has been dealt with, discuss and agree what steps to take to ensure there is no confusion or further misunderstanding in future similar situations.

14.8.3 Challenge Perceptions – Including Your Own

One way of dealing with people is to review how you perceive them. Changes to systems often take place when someone is not happy with current circumstances. If nurtured, these people could become your agents for change. Whenever you catch staff complaining about something, it is better not to listen and sympathise. A better response would be to ask them to suggest a solution. This may catch them by surprise, as they would probably not be used to such a response. They may be more used to getting people to agree and complain with them. People who are challenged to do something about the situation tend to stop complaining at the very least because what you are really saying is 'if you are not prepared to do anything about it, then stop moaning'.

14.8.4 Do Not Allow a Perpetual Complainer to Prevent Progress

If you have an idea that you want to raise with your team, it is wise to present it to each of them individually before raising it at a team meeting. Ask for their ideas and feedback. When you eventually raise the idea at a team meeting, you can ensure that most of the team will support you. If an individual realises that they are on their own with their usual negative opinions, they will be more reluctant to relay them. If they do, then ask them and the rest of the team what an alternative solution would be. Do not dwell on any negatives; focus on the positives. Always have an answer ready for the usual negative responses (see Table 14.1).

14.8.5 Holding a Negative View of Oneself

Some members of staff may consistently complain that they are not good enough. For example:

'Here is the work you asked me to do; it is not very good'.
'I went to that meeting for you, but I was useless. I am no good at that sort of thing'.
'I am too stupid/too old/not intelligent enough'.

TABLE 14.1 Sample Answers for Negative Responses Within Meetings

Negative Response	Answer
'I do not see how it will work. They will never allow us to do that'.	'Who will not allow us to do that? Why do you think that they will not allow us to? I see no reason why not'.
'It has all been tried before, and it never makes any difference'.	'Well, I am sorry it did not work out for you before, but this time it is different because…'
'It is always back to us. Why should we have to do all the work?'	'If you want to see things improve, then you have to make the effort. Complaining will achieve nothing but taking action will'.

All these sorts of comments do is demonstrate a lack of confidence. Sometimes it is done to protect them from negative feedback. If they have said it themselves, then someone else is hardly likely to say it again. If you are continuously giving all members of your staff positive feedback, then you will be very unlikely to hear these things. So, if it is happening, question your style of leadership; are you giving enough feedback (see Chapter 3)?

On the other hand, you may get the odd one or two people who will put themselves down in order to get people to tell them how wonderful they are. In this case, tell them if you did not think they were good enough they would not be part of your team, and you do not want to hear them talking like that again, and leave it at that.

14.9 STAFF WHO ARE CONTINUALLY LATE FOR DUTY

We have probably all done it; seethed in silence when a member of staff wanders into handover 5 or 10 min late. Not only that, but some even have the nerve to bring a cup of coffee in too!

14.9.1 The Problem With Lateness

Lateness can cause huge problems within a team. In many other areas of work, people have less need to start on time because their jobs are outcome focused. This means that as long as they get the job done, it does not really matter when or even where they work. But in nursing and any other jobs that involve shift work, getting to work on time has a greater importance. Arriving late results in:

- interruption and delaying of handover
- staff from the previous shift getting off late, as they have to repeat everything for the latecomers

- the latecomer risking missing vital information about their patients and therefore compromising their ability to care for the patients when the previous shift goes home
- reduced morale and working relationships within the team becoming fragmented

Ignore lateness at your peril. If allowed to continue, it may become accepted as normal practice. The staff will become divided into those that are conscientious and come in on time and those that do not. Consistent lateness is a reflection of poor attitudes about work.

14.9.2 Getting to the Root of the Matter

If you notice that a member of staff is regularly coming to work late, you should first try to uncover the underlying causes. If they are having genuine problems getting to work on time, such as their bus timetable being incompatible with shift start times, then it is better to compromise and formally agree to a later start time. That way, working practice can change in advance to accommodate this.

If you come to the conclusion that it is simply a poor attitude to work or because some staff members are not committed, then you need to consider your leadership style again:

1. Are your team working towards shared goals?
2. Do you give feedback to each member of staff every time you work with them?
3. Do you know each individual in your team well?

If you hesitated or answered no to any of the above questions, then perhaps you need to ascertain what else you can do to provide a more motivating environment first (see Chapter 3).

14.9.3 Find a Solution Together

If a member of staff continues to arrive late for duty despite you having ascertained that there are no extenuating personal circumstances and you know you have done everything outlined in Chapter 3 to maintain a motivating environment, the next step is to concentrate on finding a solution *with* them. Do not continually ask them why they are late each time. If you do, you will just receive a barrage of excuses. Turn the question round to make them suggest a solution: 'Despite our previous meeting, you still turn up late for most of your shifts. What can we do about it?'

Do not allow the rest of your staff to accommodate lateness. They must not wait to give handover. Ensure they always start on time without them. Make sure they do not summarise what the latecomer has missed. They must be made to catch up themselves afterwards. They should change, but if they do not, you have two options.

14.9.3.1 Option 1: Aim Towards the Disciplinary Process

When dealing with persistent lateness, it is essential that you keep accurate records of all episodes, including lateness from lunch breaks. You must be able to demonstrate that you have met with the staff member to determine any possible solutions and agreed actions. Make sure that during your meetings you have at some stage outlined when the lateness qualifies for disciplinary action. Before you take this route, you need to show that you have fully explored all possible solutions.

14.9.3.2 Option 2: Encourage Them to Look at Other Roles Where They Will Be Stimulated

Continual lateness, despite the actions outlined above, indicates a lack of commitment to the job so perhaps it is not the right one for them. If you have a member of staff who is truly not happy in their work, they may simply be in the wrong speciality. Do not give up on them and wait for them to leave. Help them to identify what job would really stimulate them and assist them in developing the skills to be able to apply for a post in their chosen field. Whatever happens, you do not want staff leaving your ward and telling others how they hated working in your area. Helping them to attain their chosen job will see them leave on a more positive note.

14.9.4 Prevention Is Better Than Cure

Make sure you have included in your induction package:

- what time shifts begin and what is considered late
- how to inform the rest of the team if they know they will be late
- when and how disciplinary action will be undertaken for lateness

Many organisations now have some sort of code of conduct for their employees. This usually includes the above points, so inclusion of the document in the induction package may suffice. Remember also that if you expect staff to be punctual in their arrival to work, then you should also meet their expectations of getting off work on time. Do not expect staff to stay late (unless you are paying them extra). Giving time back is insufficient compensation for people having to stay late (unpaid) regularly at work.

14.9.4.1 Action Points

- Ensure all members of staff adhere to the uniform policy. If any refuse, find out why and propose alternative solutions. Take the disciplinary route only when all other avenues have been exhausted.

- Involve all members of staff in all changes by presenting the initial problem first and asking for proposed solutions. Do not present the solution first.
- Do not allow any staff members to regularly stay behind to finish work or miss their breaks. Work with them if necessary to help develop prioritising skills.
- If you feel a member of your staff is 'lazy', find out first if there are any problems with illness, personal commitments or if it is simply a lack of motivation. Take action to increase their motivation either to work more efficiently or find another job.
- Be aware of the process to take should a member of staff turn up unfit for work through alcohol or drugs, so that the appropriate action is taken in any such event.
- Resolve any problems between members of your team by calling them to a meeting immediately and taking specific action. Do not allow any situation of conflict to continue.
- Use competency packages to improve the skills of junior team members. Encourage senior team members with poor standards to review the competency packages, thus improving their own skills in the process.
- Confront any staff members who try to manipulate you.
- Encourage your team to transform negative statements into positive solutions.
- Take action immediately to stop people being persistently late for duty or late back from breaks. Show the rest of your team that you will not tolerate lateness.
- Ensure your ward induction package includes a section on how staff members are expected to behave.

APPENDIX 14.1 EXAMPLE OF A SWOT ANALYSIS FOR BEDSIDE HANDOVER

Strengths (Internal)	Weaknesses (Internal)
Able to match names with faces	Potential problems with confidentiality
Able to scrutinise observation charts and care plans at the same time	Unable to get a chance to sit down and have a cup of tea (often only chance during shift is during handover)
Able to introduce self to patient	
Patient can be fully involved	Unable to chat/catch up with colleagues
Less time hanging around waiting for office handover to finish before being able to go home	Staff do not get to know everything about every patient
	Patients may not like it
Opportunities (external)	**Threats (external)**
New handheld computers being introduced for wards that use bedside handover	New flexible working policy affecting handover times
Complies with CQC standards	Forthcoming cutbacks in staffing

Chapter 15

Get the Best Advice

Making any decision in nursing is often a multifocal approach. It is good practice to try and not to rely on just one source of advice when making decisions. How do you know for sure that the person's advice is sound? How do you know they are giving you the best option? Trying to seek advice from a variety of sources will help you make a more informed decision based on as many facts and opinions as you can access. Try to include your team in any decision-making process when you can. Enable them to have an input and influence over the decisions you have to make which affect them.

There are various departments within healthcare trusts to which you can go for advice, some which are under-utilised by nurse managers. As a senior person within the trust you have access to solicitors, senior professional advisors, educational advisors, counselling services, human resource advisors, computer experts and many more. You should never have to make decisions or struggle with any aspects of your work without being able to access the appropriate support.

15.1 KNOW WHERE TO GO FOR LEGAL ADVICE

15.1.1 Solicitors

NHS organisations appoint solicitors to act and advise on their behalf in respect of legal issues. If you require legal advice regarding a problem that has arisen or may arise at work, most organisations have a procedure in place through which you can access these solicitors. This procedure is there to ensure that they are not being asked the same questions from different areas within the organisation. The solicitors can usually be accessed through the person who deals with litigation and claims, known as the litigation and claims manager, legal services manager or clinical governance manager.

It is advisable to locate the appropriate person within your organisation and to keep a copy of their contact details available at all times both for you and your staff. Your director of nursing should be your first port of call for any professional issues. They have more experience and may be able to advise without calling on the solicitors.

If you have an emergency out of hours, contact the duty manager who will have access. Some solicitors provide a 24-h helpline for advice on clinical issues, but this number would usually be restricted for the use of a 'named' senior manager or on-call managers. Some organisations hold contracts with solicitors who include free training for staff, which is well worth accessing, but often you will have to ask first. This service is not usually widely advertised.

If a solicitor is needed for a problem, you will be supported by the trust's legal team, who will take the lead role in the incident.

15.1.2 Trade Union Representatives

Every NHS organisation has a number of trade union representatives as well as a lead steward whose role is to protect members' rights and ensure they are treated fairly. They are specifically trained for the role. They will provide help and guidance with issues concerning employment rights, discrimination, health and safety legislation and concerns about poor practices. You can also get advice regarding legal or potential legal issues directly from your local regional office.

Both the Royal College of Nursing (RCN) and UNISON provide members with online advice services where you can get information on legal issues. These can include personal, non-work-related legal advice.

15.2 KNOW WHERE TO GO FOR PROFESSIONAL ADVICE

15.2.1 The Director of Nursing

One of the key responsibilities of your director of nursing is to provide professional leadership to all nurses and midwives within the organisation. They will provide advice personally or direct you to the appropriate place to find the information you require. If you have a non-clinical line manager and need advice on a professional matter, there is no reason why you cannot contact your director or deputy director of nursing directly. Use the phone if it is an emergency; otherwise use email. Directors of nursing may be the most senior nurses within your organisation, but they recognise that ward managers are a vital asset and will ensure you can access the appropriate professional advice and support.

Most nurse directors have at least one deputy director plus a small team of senior healthcare professionals to assist them in their corporate-wide role. The director of nursing, together with their team, provides a support system for nurses, midwives and allied health professionals to help maintain high standards of care across the organisation.

15.2.2 The Nursing and Midwifery Council

The main aim of the NMC is to ensure that registered nurses and midwives provide high standards of care and to protect the public. This is achieved by:

- maintaining the professional register;
- standards;

- investigating and dealing with allegations of misconduct;
- providing a professional advice service for nurses and midwives.

The advice service is free and confidential. It is provided by a team of professionals qualified in various specialities such as mental health nursing, paediatric nursing, adult nursing and learning disabilities. You can email or call one of the professional officers with your query or access information from their website.

In addition, you can access all current NMC publications such as *Raising and Escalating Concerns: Guidance for Nurses and Midwives* or *Guidance for Continuing Professional Development for Nurse and Midwife Prescribers.* These can all be downloaded free from their website.

15.2.3 University Lecturers

Your link lecturer is the obvious choice for advice regarding issues in your speciality, but there is no reason why you cannot access other university lecturers for expert advice. Most would be only too happy to provide information within their speciality. Email is usually the best approach to use as lecturers can be difficult to contact by phone due to their Monday to Friday working pattern and tight teaching schedules.

Keep a copy of the annual course prospectus from your local university's department of nursing studies or health and social care. This will contain all the contact details of the lecturers in each speciality. You will find most lecturers helpful in professional matters and if they do not know the answer, they will usually refer you to someone who does.

15.3 UTILISE THE CHAPLAINCY DEPARTMENT

Chaplaincy services are under-used by some ward managers. They usually offer an excellent service which involves more than just providing spiritual care to patients of various faiths. They also provide a service for staff, including those who do not profess any particular faith. The chaplaincy services can be invaluable when your team is going through a particularly hard time, such as dealing with difficult deaths or more deaths than usual. They can also be very supportive in times of staff shortages when members of your team may be distressed at being unable to meet the usual high standards of care.

15.3.1 Bereavement

Part of the role of the chaplaincy department is to educate staff in dealing with bereavement. They can also provide support to members of your team who suffer a personal bereavement. However, they will not come to you; you have to access these services in times of need. It can be difficult if you do not know them very well. It is better to prepare by building up a good relationship with your chaplaincy team; however, they are always happy to help anyone who needs their guidance and support.

15.3.2 Staff Support

It does not matter if you or members of your staff are not religious. Hospital chaplaincy services do not impose their religious beliefs. Their role is to meet both religious and spiritual needs and they are not concerned about whether or not staff members go to church.

It would be wise to include a meeting with a member of the chaplaincy service as part of your induction programme for new members of staff (if your trust-wide induction programme does not already include this).

Many occupational health departments also offer staff support services, including mental health and well-being drop-in clinics. Speak with your occupational health department to understand what they can offer to you and your team.

15.3.3 Staff Training and Development

Chaplains working in healthcare receive specialist training, education and experience in working with people in challenging situations. They can contribute to your staff training programme in a number of subjects such as:

- listening skills
- dealing with difficult situations
- appreciation of religious, cultural and linguistic diversity
- advanced directives or 'living wills'

Their skills may also be helpful in the facilitation of clinical supervision groups for your staff.

Consider inviting one of the chaplaincy team to some of your ward meetings. Their skills may be particularly useful in debriefing sessions following distressing circumstances such as serious incidents requiring investigation, accidents or mistakes.

15.3.4 Increase Staff Awareness

Make sure all members of staff are fully aware of how to access the chaplaincy service and that they do not have to be religious in order to do so. Ensure they know they can call on the chaplaincy service for advice on a range of matters including advance directives (living wills), palliative care and even personal support for individual staff, including bereavement or relationship issues. The chaplains are increasingly being used as someone to talk to who will listen and help individuals to reflect in absolute confidence. They also have the advantage in that they are not part of any internal hierarchy.

Obviously, it will be far easier to call on their advice if you have built up a good working relationship with them in the first place. This is what networking is all about. It is a major part of your role as a manager. It is best not to leave it until your chaplaincy service contacts you or when you feel in need of their help and assistance.

Chaplaincy services are available 24 h a day as an on-call service in most hospitals.

15.4 UTILISE NURSE SPECIALISTS

The role of the nurse specialist varies between organisations, but overall they tend to fall into two categories:

1. Trust-wide nurse specialists.
2. Departmental nurse specialists.

The trust-wide nurse specialists usually report directly to the nursing director and have responsibility across the organisation because their area of expertise involves a large majority, if not all, of the patients. The trust-wide specialities include areas such as infection control and tissue viability. They are responsible for implementing and maintaining standards of care and monitoring performance throughout the organisation.

The departmental nurse specialists are also responsible for standards of care within their speciality across the organisation. The difference is that their speciality involves a specific group of patients. These include areas such as diabetes, respiratory and epilepsy. Their duties usually involve managing a caseload of patients, often on an outpatient basis, where they are responsible for activities such as running clinics, performing diagnostic tests and providing follow-up care and support.

15.4.1 Different Education and Development Responsibilities

The main priority for trust-wide specialists is usually the education and development of staff. Their role is to reduce common problems such as infection and pressure sores through promotion of best practice.

The main priority for departmental nurse specialists is the provision of care for their caseload of patients. They also have a responsibility for the education and development of staff within the rest of the organisation but only as and when that can be fitted around their core responsibilities. It is not their main priority, but they will do their best to be available for specialist advice and support where possible.

15.4.2 Be Wary of De-Skilling Your Staff

It has become an issue in some areas where a nurse specialist may be called as soon as a patient within their speciality is admitted. The problem here is that nurse specialists are not employed to undertake the work that a general nurse should be quite capable of doing. If, for example, a patient is admitted to a general medical ward with angina, it should not be necessary to call in a cardiac nurse specialist to provide rehabilitation advice. That should remain within the remit of the general medical nurse.

The role of the nurse specialist is to provide appropriate education and advice to enable the general nurses to improve their own skills. If members of your team fall into the habit of calling in a nurse specialist each time, they will lose their skills in that area. Your role as ward manager is to continuously improve the skills of your team. Use the nurse specialists to help you in this role by asking them to provide education and development for your team.

Develop close links with all the trust-wide nurse specialists plus those who are directly linked with your speciality. Usually the trust-wide specialist nurses will be working towards specific targets and will be only too happy to come along at your request to assist in the education and development of staff. This also helps them in achieving their targets, as do link nurse roles.

15.4.3 Link Nurse Roles

Beware of having a link nurse role for each specialist subject. Ideally each individual in your team should have no more than one link nurse role, otherwise they may not be able to make the most of the development opportunities for each subject area and they risk becoming overloaded.

There will always be more link nurse roles than there are available nurses within your team. The key is to prioritise. Any areas linked to the quality outcome indicators should come top of the list. For example, it is advisable to have a link nurse for infection control and tissue viability. Other link nurse roles depend on the frequency of patients admitted with the specialist condition on your ward. You may find diabetes is the next key priority on a ward where a large number of patients admitted are diabetic.

If there are more link nurse roles than the number of staff in your team, get your team together and decide what your top priorities are. Make a conscious decision to leave out the rest. Inform your manager in writing (email will suffice) about the decision you have made with your team and why. You may have an outcry from nurse specialists who want a link nurse on your ward to maintain communications, but the welfare of your team comes first. Work together with them to find some other less time-consuming way that you can maintain communications.

15.5 HELP PATIENTS AND RELATIVES ACCESS THE RIGHT ADVICE

15.5.1 Patient Advice and Liaison Service

All patients and relatives have access to advice and support in making a formal complaint about their health services, but in England, the Department of

Health has gone one step further through the development of patient advice and liaison services (PALS). Every NHS organisation in England now has a PALS office employing several individuals to provide information and advice to patients and relatives about any concerns they may have while in hospital.

PALS is unique to NHS England; however, the services in Scotland, Wale and Northern Ireland work on the same principle, but are named as follows:

● Scotland – Patient Advice and Support Service (PASS)
● Wales – Community Health Council (CHC)
● Northern Ireland – Health & Social Care Board (HSC)

The main role of PALS officers is to resolve problems and concerns quickly by liaising with healthcare professionals and managers on the patients' behalf. They act as an independent body so that patients and staff feel that any complaint is investigated fairly.

It is prudent that if patients feel that an issue is not being resolved, they should be referred to PALS. This is not a sign of poor leadership and management; rather it is a sign of openness and willingness to learn from complaints. It also offers the patient or relatives making the complaint an independent person to speak with. When patients and relatives are going through a trauma, it may be difficult for them to articulate to others involved – it is important to remember no one expects to be in hospital; it is an alien place and one that often is not expected.

PALS are not only there to deal just with complaints. Often, patients and relatives will submit positive feedback to them as well. The PALS officers keep records of all visits to enable you to learn from the information.

15.5.2 Information Leaflets and Digital Support

It is imperative to ensure the supply of information sheets and leaflets is always plentiful, including those on how to make a complaint. However, given the huge array of literature which is now available, try to ensure that you and your staff select the appropriate ones for individual patients' and relatives' needs rather than expect them to help themselves. Patients who are given specific leaflets (with their name written on the front) are more likely to read and take note than if they were just left to help themselves from the leaflet rack. It is also important to direct patients to digital support. Much of the information found on leaflets is now easily accessible online, via a mobile device or computer/tablet device. Many information services also offer 'apps' to help people manage their condition better. The NHS website has a wide variety of apps that it has approved; it would be good to familiarise yourself with these and promote them to your patients.

15.5.3 Ward Rounds

Some patients and relatives become completely 'tongue-tied' when confronted with a group of doctors standing around the bedside. It is one of the main reasons why a patient's nurse should be part of the ward round. The nurse's role is to act as the patient's advocate, encouraging them to ask questions or asking on their behalf if necessary.

Your staff should routinely advise patients and relatives to prepare for ward rounds and other visits by writing down their questions in advance. They should be reassured that this is normal and that the doctor (or other healthcare professional) would prefer this to ensure that the patients' needs have been met. Illness makes patients and relatives a lot more vulnerable than they would be normally. Do not expect them to be able to access all the right information by themselves.

If after the ward round patients and relatives still have questions, ask them to write them down. If possible, try and get them answered by the medical team as soon as possible, or ensure that before ward round commences, the medical team is aware the patient would like these questions reviewed.

15.6 KEEP UP-TO-DATE WITH RISK MANAGEMENT ISSUES

Risk management basically means taking measures to reduce the likelihood of any harm happening to your patients and staff. Managing healthcare delivery will always involve a degree of risk, but minimising those risks is a key part of your role. The use of incident reporting forms will help monitor the trends of situations posing risks. It would be prudent to publish your top three risks for your department so that your staff are more aware and can offer solutions.

15.6.1 Performance Indicators for Risk Management

Your organisation will have a set of performance indicators to measure the effectiveness in the way they identify, reduce and manage risk. The main NHS performance indicators are set nationally and vary according to whether you are in England, Wales, Scotland or Northern Ireland. In England, the NHS Resolution team (NHSR) has specific risk management standards against which your trust is assessed (NHSR, 2018).

It is important that you are aware of your organisation's targets for minimising risk and that your staff are trained in risk management. You should also access training for yourself in incident investigation and root cause analysis, if you have not already done so.

15.6.2 Risk Management Board

The chief executive has overall responsibility for meeting the statutory requirements and guidance issued by the Department of Health. Most healthcare organisations have a risk management board and employ a specific team of staff to ensure that you have access to the right advice and support. They also ensure the appropriate policies and procedures are in place to help you minimise clinical and non-clinical risk. Find out who is responsible for clinical governance or risk management within your organisation and make sure they become part of your network. Perhaps even shadow them for a day. Not only will you benefit from their knowledge and find out what you should be doing, but also you will get to know them well enough to be able to call on them for expert advice when required. You will also get to know their team and which individuals are the best to call for advice and support.

15.6.3 Directorate Risk Management Committee

Your directorate will also have a specific group or committee which continually assesses and manages risk. This could be part of your directorate clinical governance group or you may have a separate directorate risk management group. It would be advisable to make sure you are a member of this group.

Be careful if you decide to delegate the role of risk management to a member of your team. You still remain accountable for ensuring that effective risk management measures are undertaken in your ward or department. It is advisable that you retain the role of risk management lead for your area and ensure you get regular feedback from your link staff for issues such as manual handling and health and safety. You retain overall responsibility for all risk management issues so make sure you are kept well informed to be able to ensure your systems and processes are all in order.

15.7 CONSULT POLICIES, PROCEDURES AND GUIDELINES

15.7.1 Why So Many Policies?

It seems that there are policies and procedures for everything we do these days, including of course a policy for the storage and filing of policies! But looking at it positively, the more policies and procedures that your organisation has is indicative of how well employees are looked after and valued.

Policies and procedures are very important in informing your day-to-day work. They indicate what the organisation expects with regard to staff behaviour and work standards. They guide you as to what is acceptable and what is not. Without this guidance, you would have no standard with which to measure others. If members of staff produce a lower standard of work, there would be little you could do about it without the appropriate policy or procedure in place. You and your staff would also have fewer rights. For the majority of questions you will ever have within your role, the majority of answers will be found in a policy or procedure.

15.7.2 Accessibility

Policies and procedures are useful documents and should be easily accessible on your intranet system for all staff to consult during the course of their shift.

They can often be a better source of advice than seeking someone else's opinion. They not only outline good practice, but they also include the most current legislation. Try to read the appropriate policy regarding any staff management issues before consulting other individuals for advice. Policies and procedures give you a good idea about the correct line of action to follow in most situations.

15.7.3 Communication of Policy Changes

Whenever you receive a new, revised or updated policy, find out exactly what has been changed in the policy. You can do this by calling the person responsible for the revised policy or procedure. Once you have done this, inform all your staff. If you just tell your staff that the policy has been replaced with a new one, it is highly unlikely that anyone will have the time or inclination to read it through. However, they will take note if you highlight what the changes are either in your ward communication book or via a team meeting. Asking staff to read through whole policies and procedures is unrealistic; highlighting the changes will ensure that staff are kept up to date.

15.7.4 Evidence-Based Guidelines

Ensure that evidence-based guidelines and standards are also easily accessible for your team. All clinical guidelines you use on your ward should be based on the best possible evidence. Guidelines should not just be an outline of the current practice on your ward for new members. You must make sure they are up to date.

However, updating guidelines takes valuable time, which you and your team probably do not have. Try and use your specialist association for guidelines pertaining to your speciality and use national guidelines wherever possible. *The Royal Marsden Manual of Clinical Procedures* is an ideal example of evidence-based guidelines which are applicable for use in most areas (Dougherty and Lister, 2015). Many organisations now have this available online but, if not, it is worth having a book like this available on the ward for your staff. It will save you and your staff wasting time on having to develop your own and continually having to update them.

The National Institute for Health and Clinical Excellence (NICE) guidelines are also easily accessible online and the Scottish Intercollegiate Guidelines Network (SIGN) guidelines are available in Scotland. Both sets of guidelines are accessible for all healthcare professionals both in and outside the United Kingdom.

If you are really keen on developing your own, get the right help and support. Contact your organisation's practice development department. If they do not have the right expertise, they will still be able to help by finding the right person or the right information on your behalf. They will also be able to advise on how to formulate the guidelines and standards and how to get them validated.

15.8 MAXIMISE COMPUTER ACCESS

15.8.1 The Internet

Nothing beats the Internet for providing instant access to information. It means that individuals do not have to leave the ward area to find the information they need to enhance their practice. There are many websites that you can access for up-to-date clinical information. If you are using these websites for evidenced-based information, make sure they are of credible sources, such as National institute of clinical and healthcare Excellence (NICE), British National Formulary (BNF), etc.

If advising patients to access information, ensure they go via NHS choices to get patient appropriate advice.

Many professional bodies, such as the RCN, have extensive online libraries of articles and information that can be accessed online as well.

If looking for evidence outside of national and NHS webpages, ensure that you use credible sources, such as Elsevier for scientific papers.

15.8.2 Getting Your Staff to Use Computers

Some nurses are still 'computer shy' and find it difficult to use computers. Try and encourage the more IT literate members of your team to help and teach those who are less so. There are also various IT courses that staff can access. All staff (including those with good IT skills) should attend regular computer skills training not only to keep abreast of all the new IT systems being introduced, but more importantly to maintain awareness of regulations regarding the handling of confidential information, particularly with the increasing computerisation of patient records.

In addition, you should ensure there are enough computers on your ward so that one is available at all times for staff to look up information instantly without having to queue.

15.9 UTILISE THE KNOWLEDGE AND SKILLS OF YOUR NURSING COLLEAGUES

15.9.1 Channel the Enthusiasm Within Your Team

As pointed out in Chapter 3, a good leader knows the strengths and weaknesses of all their team members. Work on those strengths. It you have an issue where you need more knowledge in order to make an informed decision, delegating the task of fact finding is often useful for the development of one of the individuals within your team. Do not delegate unless it serves a useful purpose for the person you are delegating to. Your junior sister/charge nurses need as much experience as they can get to prepare them for the next role. Make sure you learn together with each new experience.

15.9.2 Make Finding Information a Staff Development Opportunity

If you come across a problem which you have never dealt with before, getting others to find out what the options are for dealing with the problem can be good experience for them as well as helping you. Do not always assume that if you do not know what to do; it is up to you to find out. You can still ask others to find out for you. There may be someone in your team that actually knows the answer already; utilise the skills around you.

Whenever you are confronted with staff members who have a problem, be honest: 'I have no idea what to do in this situation. Who do you think might be able to help? Try calling them to see what they advise'. It is important to remember, although you may be the most senior member of staff on your ward/unit at the time, there is always someone more senior than you to ask for advice, 24 h a day. Whether this is someone as close as your own line manager, or the on-call tier team, there will always be someone who can offer support and advice.

15.9.3 Draw on the Experience of Your Peers

Regularly meeting with other ward managers within your organisation is one way of learning from them, but it is also a good idea to set up some sort of network in between these meetings. This ensures that you have instant access to their knowledge and experience. Email is often the best way to do this. If you have not already done so, set up a group email address of all the ward managers within your organisation and encourage them to do the same. This can prove invaluable in cases where you need urgent information. Few ward managers with the appropriate knowledge would ignore the following email addressed to the group: 'A member of staff has come to me with an allegation of bullying from one of the agency nurses. I have not dealt with this situation before. If anyone else has experience of a similar issue, I would be grateful to know how you handled it'.

Always remember to remain confidential and never divulge sensitive information which could result in the individuals involved being identified. You can contact each other by phone or face-to-face afterwards if details need to be discussed in depth.

15.9.4 Use Email

All the ward managers within your organisation would benefit by maintaining close contact and learning from each other's experiences. In the past, without email, this has been difficult because of the nature of the role. Most would be reluctant to call colleagues and interrupt their work and you do not have time to keep leaving the ward to go around and talk to your colleagues. With email, you do not have to leave the ward and you are not interrupting your colleagues in the course of their work. In addition, email takes up far less time and is a lot more succinct.

If you are not keeping a constant dialogue with your colleagues in this manner, you could be losing out on an extremely useful source of advice. There is nothing to stop you starting an email dialogue through the group address system. Contact your organisation's IT department for further ideas, which could include having your own ward manager's webpage based on frequently asked questions or even a discussion forum. A little time invested at the beginning goes a long way in terms of help and support in the future.

15.10 UTILISE THE PRACTICE DEVELOPMENT TEAM

Most healthcare organisations have some sort of professional or practice development team. They are usually directly managed and report to the director or deputy director of nursing. Their role is to work with all members of the healthcare team but particularly with ward managers, to facilitate improvements in clinical practice and spread good practice across the organisation. They support and advise all healthcare professionals and provide education and development not accessed through the universities (although they often link closely with local academic institutions).

The work of the practice development teams usually involves the following:

- Development and implementation of policies, procedures and best practice guidelines based on evidence.
- Provision of mandatory training, student and healthcare assistant (HCA) support and further clinical training.
- Dissemination of examples of good practice across the organisation.
- Assistance for staff to learn and take action from their experiences and patient feedback (e.g. from the complaints process).
- Improving staff access to the best evidence.

Try to involve the practice development team in any issue that involves changing or improving practice. If they are unable to give appropriate advice themselves, they will facilitate access to others who can. Some issues can be quite controversial, such as nil-by-mouth policies or nurse prescribing. The practice development team will help and guide you throughout the process. Even if you do not feel confident in the skills of your practice development team, it is best to keep them informed of any changes and improvements in your area to avoid duplication of any work in other departments. They can also be an invaluable source of information. The team usually includes at least the following members.

Some specialised clinical areas, such as intensive care areas, may not utilise the hospital professional development team the way other teams do. If you have a specialised unit area, ensure that your practice development team still liaises with the rest of the hospital's teams. Although the skill set may be very different, teaching principles and hospital policies and procedures will still be reviewed and be relevant to you areas.

15.10.1 Practice Placement Facilitator and Practice Educators

These people are usually employed in part or fully by the local universities to ensure that student nurses have appropriate placements and support during those placements. If you have any problems with students or problems with too many or too few students, these people should be your first port of call. Practice educators, however, are not just for students; they can help with developing newly qualified nurses or new to speciality areas. They can also offer ongoing refresher education to all members of staff.

15.10.2 A Healthcare Assistant Coordinator

An HCA coordinator is usually responsible for overseeing the training and development of HCAs throughout the organisation. They will also have links with external organisations/universities that deliver the diploma level two and three education programmes for HCAs.

15.10.3 A Training and Development Coordinator

This person is usually responsible for coordinating the contracts with the local academic institutions and private education providers. Sometimes this role is incorporated into the deputy director of nursing role.

Nurses are also brought into the practice development team on secondments to facilitate the implementation of various national projects such as the Productive Series, safeguarding of vulnerable adults or dementia awareness. Together the team can be an invaluable source of advice and support. It is up to you to build up a good working relationship so you can call on them for advice in future situations.

15.10.3.1 Action Points

- Find out how to contact your organisation's solicitors both during and out of hours. Keep the details available in your ward office should the need arise.
- Find out who the main union officials are in your organisation; get to know them and add them to your network.
- Locate a copy of the course directory from your local university on the ward, so that you can access lecturers/experts in various subjects if required.
- Get to know your chaplaincy lead, add them to your network and ensure that all new recruits meet with them during their induction programme.
- Review the link nurse roles to ensure that each member of your team has no more than one. If necessary, prioritise with your team and set up different modes of communication to receive the necessary specialist information.
- Review your team's use of PALS and look for ways of improving the service you provide at ward level via appropriate information leaflets and staff education.

- Find out and familiarise yourself with *all* your organisation's performance indicators.
- Review all the policies and procedures on your ward, making sure they are up-to-date and easily accessible for all your staff.
- Take steps to ensure all members of your team are IT literate and make the most of resources available.
- Set up a group email address on your computer to include all other ward managers within your organisation for access to support and advice.
- Get to know your practice development team and include them within your professional network.

REFERENCES

NHS Resolution. 2018. NHS Indemnity: Arrangements for Clinical Negligence Claims in the NHS. NHS Resolution. London.

Dougherty, L., Lister, S., 2015. Royal Marsden Hospital Manual of Clinical Nursing Procedures: Professional Edtion. 9e Oxford, Wiley-Blackwell.

Index

(*Note:* Page numbers followed by "f" indicate figures, "t" indicate tables.)